The Long Road to Sleep
info@longroadtosleep.com

2nd Edition
June 2020

The author of this material makes no medical claims for its use. This material is not intended to treat, diagnose nor cure any illness. If you need medical attention, please consult your doctor. This book is not intended as a substitute for the medical advice of physicians. The reader should regularly consult a physician in matters relating to his/her health and particularly with respect to any symptoms that may require diagnosis or medical attention.

You must consult your doctor or health care professional before making any changes to the prescribed medicine you are taking. If you are pregnant or nursing, or if you are elderly, or if you have a chronic or recurring condition other than insomnia, I highly recommend you contact your doctor before embarking on any suggestions or ideas provided in this book.

Any application of the techniques, ideas, and suggestions here are at the reader's sole discretion and risk. The author expressly disclaims responsibility for any adverse effects from following this advice.

No responsibility or liability is assumed by the author for any injury, damage or financial loss sustained to person or property from the use of this information, personal or otherwise, either directly or indirectly. While every effort has been made to ensure reliability and accuracy of the information within, all liability, negligence or otherwise, from any use, misuse or abuse of the operation of any methods, strategies, instructions or ideas contained in the material herein, is the sole responsibility of the reader.

# The Long Road to Sleep

## How I Overcame Decades of Sleep Maintenance Insomnia

Paul Linsell

# Acknowledgements

This book has been born out of the frustration of dealing with insomnia for so long, and it wouldn't have been possible without the support of my family. I'd also like to thank Chris Ashbrook and Harry Linsell for their help with proof-reading and editing the book.

I'd also like to thank Dr. James L. Wilson, Deborah Maragopoulos MN FNP, Square One Publishers, Inc. and Hammersmith Health Books for graciously granting me permission to cite excerpts from their books.

# Contents

# The Long Road to Sleep

## Introduction

When I first considered writing this book, I thought, who am I to be writing a book about sleep? I'm not a doctor. I'm not any kind of health care professional. I'm just a regular guy, an ordinary man in the street. But I have battled and suffered with chronic insomnia for over 30 years. As a result, I know insomnia very well. I know the despair and desperation. Insomnia is a relentless, unforgiving and cruel curse. It's like living with a malicious, fire-breathing dragon permanently perched on your shoulder, dragging your life down and making everything seem like a herculean effort. It can turn you into a zombie, dashing any hopes of achieving your life goals. Yet it's incredibly common in this stressful modern age and claims many victims, either from fatigue related accidents, or even suicide.

I tried just about every cure you can possibly imagine. You name it, I've pretty much tried it, everything, from consultations with top sleep specialists and a whole range of hopeful solutions, from prescription drugs to hypnotherapy, to binaural beats and a plethora of non-prescription and herbal remedies. All of which failed to fix my sleep, and all of which you'll soon read about in the following chapters.

I also consistently failed with the whole 'just letting go' thing with the psychology of sleep, and how to get off the anxiety merry-go-round. It's all very sound advice, usually given in most books about resolving insomnia and in various cognitive behaviour therapy courses, but it always seemed like I was just trying to fool myself. It was hard to just let go of the problem when I was feeling so lousy all the time. It was like going along tra la la la la, there is no insomnia, everything is peachy, just get on with my life and ignore it, it's all good. But for me, absolutely nothing changed. I still felt lousy and my sleep was still broken. I don't know, maybe some people can do that, but I just completely failed at letting go.

But, dear reader, – and this is a massive but – I have, at last, broken the cycle. Finally, I've managed to resolve decades of broken sleep. I found some things that work, when everything else had failed. Now I want to get the message out there to all you fellow sufferers. There is a small proviso, but it shouldn't make any difference. Most books and courses focus predominantly on sleep onset insomnia (getting to sleep), with little or no focus on sleep maintenance insomnia (sleeping through the night). Well I'm here to change that, hence my reason for writing this book.

My aim with this book is to make it as practical as possible, with guidance on exactly what I tried, what worked for me, and why. The book is relatively short as I try to get straight to the point without waffling on too much. And I'm not going to fill it with pages describing various sleeping problems. So this book doesn't cover specific conditions such as obstructive sleep apnoea, upper airway resistance syndrome, periodic limb movement disorder, restless leg syndrome, narcolepsy, and REM sleep behaviour disorder. But rather I focus on insomnia - sleep maintenance insomnia in particular.

I'm also not going to subject you to a chapter on why sleep is so important. Every book seems to go on into great detail about how sleep affects your health and why it's so important. That's all very informative, but for a chronic insomniac, it's just depressing to read and adds to the stress of the problem. We know sleep is important. We just want real practical help, help that actually works. If this is the first book you've read about sleep, then I'm genuinely shocked you haven't read tonnes more and I'm honoured that you've chosen this book - thank you.

# Chapter 1

## My Story

As I alluded to in the introduction, I know insomnia very well. I know its many shapes and forms and its insidious nature. I know the despair and dark thoughts that can cloud your mind night after a torturous night. I know the continual burn behind the eyes and the seemingly never-ending stream of headaches. It's like you're living your life in some kind of minimal power-save-mode and after decades of poor sleep you eventually get to the point where you no longer fear death. In fact you await its cold embrace because you might finally be able to get some decent shut-eye. So, dear reader, you have my genuine sympathy and understanding as a fellow sufferer.

Normal sleepers don't really understand and probably think it can't be that bad. They often make helpful suggestions, such as trying a warm glass of milk before bed, or a chamomile tea – because things like that help them sleep like a baby. Yeah, like that's going to magically cure decades of broken sleep. Or they say how they sleep like a log as soon as their head hits the pillow. Or they'll describe how bad their night was last week. Yeah, how awful. Try three solid decades. But you just don't have the energy to respond. So you soon learn to keep quiet about sleep, because the responses are rarely helpful or sympathetic.

Imagine you have to catch an early flight out from Heathrow and you have to get up at like 3am. Now imagine that feeling being your default, and pretty much continuous life experience. You never ever stop feeling overwhelmingly tired. That's probably the best way I can describe it to a normal sleeper. But even that doesn't really do it justice, because year after year, you start to get a cumulative negative effect that impacts your health and well-being.

I probably don't need to say much more about how bad it can be. I'm sure you bought this book because you're looking for answers, which means that just for once I'm preaching to the choir. But allow me a brief moment to describe my history and the reason for this book, a book that I like to think is different from all the other sleep books out there, many of which are filled with pages and pages of detailed information about sleep issues, yet fail to provide an effective answer.

I suffered from poor sleep for more than 30 years. Even in childhood I remember regularly lying awake for ages each night and just generally didn't sleep well. I don't even know when it started. I just know it was a permanent fixture of my life, with some years being particularly bad. I have never had a problem getting to sleep; I had trouble staying asleep, usually waking after just a few hours and then being unable to get back to sleep, sometimes for the rest of the night. Specifically, my problem has been with 'Sleep Maintenance,' a type of insomnia that's very hard to control, but that many people suffer from.

As I'm sure you're aware, this can be very deceiving, because while you might manage to actually fall asleep and sleep for a couple of hours, it's nowhere near enough. I used to go bed around 11pm and fall asleep quickly, but would be awake again by around 1 or 2am. I would then lie awake for about an hour, eventually getting out of bed, so that I could start again, so to speak. But when I did go back to bed, it was usually very difficult to fall asleep again, and I was often still awake at 5:30am. Although I was exhausted, sleep just wouldn't come. I might be able to nod off again at 6:00am, but it would be more like dozing.

I'd need to be up at 7:00am to do the school run, then go to work, or other commitments. Yet by 9:00am I was feeling ready for sleep again. Of course, I couldn't; I had the whole day ahead of me. So with energy levels crashing, I'd reach for caffeine and sugary snacks to keep me going. But it was never enough. Sometimes I'd nod off in front of my computer. My head would flop forward and I'd jolt awake. This would take the edge off the tiredness for a very short time, but I'd usually get a headache.

More often than not, I'd nap in my car during lunch break. Then I'd nap again when I got home at 5:30pm. I remember being so sleepy some days, I couldn't even talk properly. I struggled to form words. It was almost like being drunk. And

I couldn't remember things that people had said to me. Brain fog was a constant problem. Basically, I was struggling to get through each day.

Over the years, I spent well over £10,000 on specialist consultants, various therapies and treatments, not to mention all manner of pills and herbal remedies, most of which had no effect whatsoever, either positive or negative. I'm sure they must have been doing something, but I simply didn't notice any effect. I would always seem to be in minority of people for which the 'tried-and-tested' treatments didn't work. I'd read the reviews of yet another product on Amazon, with many people saying they slept so much better. And so I'd eagerly try another product which had had good reviews. But sadly, 9 times out of 10 it would have absolutely no effect... nothing, zip, nada. I'm not just talking about trying it one night and giving up. I mean sticking religiously with the whole course for several weeks. I'd be looking at the product, thinking, well that was another waste money, and wondering, what the hell is actually wrong with me? Even specialist sleep consultants admitted that my type of insomnia is one of the hardest to treat, at which point they'd reach for the prescription pad.

I'd read book after book about sleep and, again did everything they suggest, even buying the products they recommended. But alas, I only ever seem to achieve very limited improvements, if any. But all the books I've found seem to focus predominantly on sleep onset insomnia, where getting to sleep when first going to bed is the issue, with little or no mention of dealing specifically with sleep maintenance insomnia, where staying asleep is the issue.

I've even had a full-blown sleep analysis conducted, which, in itself is stressful – and it didn't help. Unfortunately all the equipment and wires stuck to me wasn't exactly conducive to sleep, so my night was even worse than usual and not typical to how I'd usually sleep. That the results showed I only slept a little, didn't really help, and in my particular case, only told me what I already knew.

I've been to see my GP on several occasions, but having already tried, or already doing everything they'd suggested, they would inevitably print off a prescription for prescription-only medication. The different drugs I was prescribed did actually have an effect – for a while. But ultimately ended up making things worse, which I'll get onto later in the book.

So several years back, during some particularly dark and challenging times from lack of sleep, I started to systematically track and note down all the things that I'd tried and whether they'd had any effect, positive or negative. And I did eventually find some lasting improvements, which is why I wrote this book. I finally discovered how to get much better sleep and altogether better life experience. This curse really can be conquered and the dragon eventually tamed. It never quite goes away completely, and does try to rear its ugly head from time to time, given half the chance, but it can be improved to the point where it's no longer life-destroying, but rather life-energising.

# Keeping Track

My sleep was always very variable, one night I might only get 3-hours sleep and then the next night I'd get 5-hours, but I'd very rarely get 6-hours, for example:

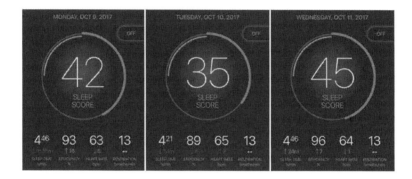

This kind of limited, erratic sleep is fine if it's for a short period of time, but my challenge was living with this amount of sleep for the rest of my life. It is certainly survivable and may even be enough for some people, but didn't seem like nearly enough for me, as you can probably tell from my introduction. Your lack of sleep may be a lot worse than mine was. If so, I sincerely sympathise with your plight and I really hope this book can help.

Nowadays, I'm consistently above 6 and half hours and usually get around 7 hours sleep, which is worlds apart from where I was, and is literally like getting my life back. Realistically based on my long history of sleep problems I probably can't achieve even better sleep than this. The elusive 8 hours may be beyond what I'm capable of. But the important thing is that I'm consistently sleeping much better than ever before and most importantly feel so much better.

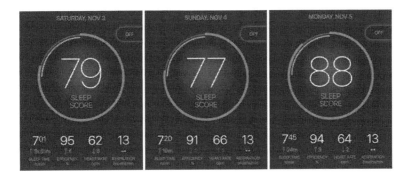

In terms of sleep tracking, I've been using the Apple Beddit 3 Sleep Monitoring device (https://www.apple.com/uk/shop/product/MUFM2B/A/beddit-sleep-monitor) and the accompanying smart phone app to track my sleep. I've tried a number of different devices and apps over the years and have found the Beddit 3 device to be pretty accurate at tracking sleep and it's completely unnoticeable, which is important. I just go to bed as normal and the app starts tracking automatically without me having to do anything. I don't feel the device is there on the mattress, no matter how much I move around or which position I sleep in. Here's an example snapshot with annotations:

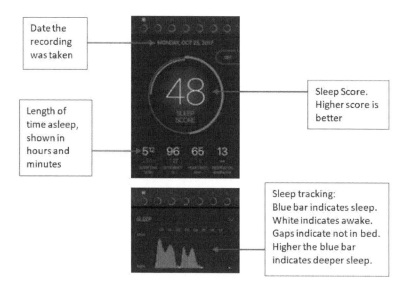

Date the recording was taken

Length of time asleep, shown in hours and minutes

Sleep Score. Higher score is better

Sleep tracking: Blue bar indicates sleep. White indicates awake. Gaps indicate not in bed. Higher the blue bar indicates deeper sleep.

Just to reiterate before we begin... I am not a doctor. I am not a sleep specialist. I'm not any kind of healthcare professional and I have absolutely no medical related training whatsoever. This book is in no way a substitute for real professional medical help, particularly if it's likely you have sleep apnoea, or some other physical related problem. The aim of this book is purely to share my own personal experience in battling decades of sleep maintenance insomnia and to provide a step by step guide as to what worked for me. I can only give you anecdotal evidence of what worked for me, with absolutely no scientific rigour whatsoever. But I've tried many 100s of different things and spent many thousands, so I sincerely hope that some of the things that have helped me, can also provide improvements for you.

# Chapter 2

## Medication

Many of the books on sleep cover in great detail the prescription drugs and over-the-counter medication you can buy, all of which make wild claims to help you sleep. It still annoys me to see these products advertised on television, as if they've finally found a cure for insomnia, when in truth, they're no more effective than a cup of warm milk. Over the years, I've tried many of these, and because none of them provided an answer, I feel that I should cover them in this book.

The sections below lists all the various products, supplements, herbal remedies, pills, treatments and other related things I've tried in order to help improve the quality and length of my sleep, the vast majority of which had little or not affect.

# Prescription Medication

## Amitriptyline 10mg

My GP prescribed Amitriptyline. I started taking 1 tablet each evening at around 9:00pm, which is about 2 hours before I sleep. Taking 1 Amitriptyline 10mg tablet worked well for me initially, and I was able to get approximately 1 hour extra sleep each night, which made a big difference to me. However, after 20 days my body built up a tolerance and the tablets were no longer effective.

I didn't want to risk taking a higher dose of Amitriptyline because of the alarming list of side-effects, and because I'd probably just build up a tolerance again, and then need yet a higher dose.

Common side-effects of Amitriptyline can include things such as: constipation, diarrhea; nausea, vomiting, upset stomach; mouth pain, unusual taste, black tongue; appetite or weight changes; urinating less than usual; itching or rash; breast swelling (in men or women); decreased sex drive, impotence, or difficulty having an orgasm!

Thankfully, just taking 1 tablet didn't cause any noticeable side effects for me. The big problem was that my sleep became worse than it was originally when I stopped the medication. As Amitriptyline only offers very limited relief, I wouldn't recommend getting sucked into trying it, at least until you've thoroughly tried all the recommendations in this book.

### Mirtazapine orodispersible 7.5mg

I was prescribed Mirtazapine after an initial consultation with a private London based sleep specialist. Rather worryingly, this was his first suggestion before trying anything else. I only took 1/2 tablet (7.5mg) each evening at around 10:00pm, which is about 1 hour before I sleep.

I did notice some improved sleep initially, but as with the Amitriptyline, my body soon built up a tolerance (albeit for the relatively low dose). I also experienced some restless leg type side effects when going to bed, and sometimes felt a little dizzy and nauseous the next day. The Magnesium body spray mentioned below helped to prevent the restless leg type side effects. But, as with the Amitriptyline, I'd recommend steering clear of prescription medication until thoroughly trying the other recommendations.

### Trazodone 50mg capsules

After Mirtazapine failed to live up to its promise in my particular case, the sleep consultant then asked me to stop the Mirtazapine for 5 days and switch to trying Trazodone. Unfortunately I didn't notice any improvement to my sleep, but seemed to get more headaches while on Trazodone.

All the chopping and changing of prescription medications generally had a negative effect and set my sleep back to being worse than it was originally. In hindsight, I'd steer clear of prescription medication for sleep.

# Non-prescription Pills, Herbal Remedies and Other Products

### Dreamy Night Time Drink

http://allrecipes.co.uk/recipe/624/dreamy-nighttime-drink.aspx

Zero improvement in sleep. No noticeable effect.

### Horlicks Original Malt Drink

https://www.amazon.co.uk/Horlicks-Original-Malt-2kg/dp/B00OD0RAMY

Zero improvement in sleep. No noticeable effect.

### Twinings Pure Camomile Tea

https://www.amazon.co.uk/Twinings-Pure-Camomile-Tea-Bags/dp/B017IYEZJM

Zero improvement in sleep. No noticeable effect.

### Kava Kava Liquid Drops 500mg (2oz) 60ml

https://www.biovea.com/uk/product_detail.aspx?pid=21523

According to the Wikipedia page about Kava (June 2020):

*"The root of the plant is used to produce a drink with sedative, anesthetic, and euphoriant properties. Its active ingredients are called kavalactones. A systematic review done by the British nonprofit Cochrane concluded it was likely to be more effective than placebo at treating short-term anxiety."*

I tried the liquid drops every day for 3 weeks. I mixed 30 drops into a small glass of water each morning and each evening before bed. The taste was slightly odd, but not unpleasant. Unfortunately, I didn't notice any improvement in my sleep. However I did seem to have vivid dreams after taking Kava Kava, which is interesting as I rarely seem to dream, or rarely remember having dreams.

### Kava Kava 500mg 60 Vegetarian Capsules

https://www.biovea.com/uk/product_detail.aspx?pid=21519

Zero improvement in sleep. No noticeable effect.
The liquid form of Kava Kava seemed to be more potent.

To learn more about Kava Kava I recommend reading Dr. Jacob Teitelbaum's book: *"From Fatigued to Fantastic: A Clinically Proven Program to Regain Vibrant Health and Overcome Chronic Fatigue and Fibromyalgia"*.

### Valerian Herbal Tincture 50ml

Zero improvement in sleep. No noticeable effect.

### Hion Dream Powder

https://www.amazon.co.uk/gp/product/B01M3R25PB

On their product page on Amazon it's noted as the world's first pure night-time super food - 14 outstanding pure & effective ingredients designed to infuse the body & mind helping you sleep deeply.

Ingredients:
- Amchur Mango
- Turmeric
- Orange Peel
- Pumpkin Seed Protein

- Goji Berry
- Baobab
- Ashwagandha
- Ginger
- Flaxseed
- Clove Powder
- Ceylon Cinnamon
- Montmorency Cherry
- Griffonia Seed Extract (5-HTP - 41mg per 5g serving)
- Sweetener: Steviol Glycosides

It's a good quality product and I'm sure must have done some good, but despite trying this for 3 solid months I didn't experience any improvements in sleep. No noticeable effects whatsoever.

**Sominex Tablets**
I did notice I was able to sleep very slightly better, but it's advisable that they're not to be used for more than 7 days. So it's not really worth it. And again you then have potential issues when stopping the tablets. You also need to be careful not to take the Sominex tablets together with any other antihistamine tablets, for example if you're taking something for hay fever or other allergies.

**Activation Products Magnesium Ease 250ml - Body Spray**
https://www.amazon.co.uk/gp/product/B01C45GGZG
Interestingly, this is one of the first things Shawn Stevenson recommends in his book *"Sleep Smarter: 21 Essential Strategies to Sleep Your Way to a Better Body, Better Health, and Bigger Success"*.

And Magnesium supplements were the first thing recommended to me by a nutritionist, so I had some hopes, but despite trying for 2-months I experienced no noticeable improvements in sleep. However this product was helpful at preventing the restless legs type side effect that could sometimes occur when taking the Mirtazapine.

I did notice that this product has now more than doubled in price from when I purchased it a year ago, which seems quite steep for seemingly very little benefit.

There are many alternative magnesium body spray products available at much more reasonable prices, however some of them are much more oily and have to be washed off the body after 20 minutes or so. This is a lot less convenient than the non-greasy type, so is something to be aware of if you're looking into trying a magnesium body spray.

**Hemp Oil Drops 5% 500mg**
Cannabidiol - also known as CBD - is one of the main cannabinoids in the cannabis plant. Cannabinoids interact with your endocannabinoid system, which helps your body maintain a state of balance and stability, or homeostasis.

Marketed as a natural anti inflammatory, it reduces pain, anxiety and stress; and helps with sleep, mood, skin. This all sounds very promising, but I didn't notice any improvements in sleep.

## 5-HTP 200mg - Double Strength 5 HTP with Added Chamomile by Puretality

https://www.amazon.co.uk/gp/product/B01IHYAMK8

Ingredients:
- 5-HTP (from 16:1 extract) - 200mg
- Chamomile - 50mg

According to Wikipedia (June 2020):

> *"5-Hydroxytryptophan (5-HTP), also known as oxitriptan, is a naturally occurring amino acid and chemical precursor as well as a metabolic intermediate in the biosynthesis of the neurotransmitter serotonin.*
>
> *5-HTP is sold over the counter in the United States, Canada, the Netherlands, and the United Kingdom as a dietary supplement for use as an antidepressant, appetite suppressant, and sleep aid. It is also marketed in many European countries for the indication of major depression under the trade names Cincofarm, Levothym, Levotonine, Oxyfan, Telesol, Tript-OH, and Triptum."*

There are many 5-HTP supplements available of vary strengths and sometimes with additional sleep-aid ingredients. They're usually marketed as a strong sleep aid, and seem to have a lot of positive reviews. However for me personally there were no improvements in sleep. Perhaps I needed to try a higher strength tablet before being able to notice any effect, but at the level I tried I experienced no noticeable benefits.

To learn more about 5-HTP I recommend reading Dr. Jacob Teitelbaum's book: *"From Fatigued to Fantastic: A Clinically*

*Proven Program to Regain Vibrant Health and Overcome Chronic Fatigue and Fibromyalgia"*.

## Vitafusion Melatonin Gummies
Vitafusion Sleep Well for Adults. Sugar Free White Tea with Passion Fruit - 60 Gummies

Ingredients:
- Melatonin - 3mg
- Passion Flower 4:1 Extract - 4.25mg
- Chamomile Flower 4:1 Extract - 4.25mg
- Lemon Balm Leaf 4:1 Extract - 4mg

I was slightly worried about taking a hormone based supplement so I started by taking just half a dose before bed and another half when waking in the night, but actually it was helpful for getting back to sleep and especially helpful when adjusting to a new time zone. I still woke very early but it did seem to help with getting back to sleep at night which is a big plus point.

Unfortunately I noticed this product is no longer available in the UK. This is due to melatonin based medication now being available only on prescription in the UK. However there are many different melatonin products available in the US, some with up to 12mg strength.

Supplementing with melatonin can be helpful particularly if you have a low-functioning thyroid, which I'll cover later in this book. But I'd recommend being cautious about using melatonin and to definitely seek advice from your GP and/or a nutritionist before proceeding with it. Side-effects are a possibility, as with all medication, but it's worth looking into melatonin along with the other recommendations in this book.

**Enzymatic Revitalizing Sleep Formula**
https://www.amazon.co.uk/gp/product/B00009M8II
Enzymatic Therapy Fatigued To Fantastic - Revitalizing Sleep Formula, 30 Caps - by NUTRILIFE

Ingredients:
- Valerian Root Extract 200mg
- Passion Flower Leaf and Flower Extract 90mg
- 5-HTP (L-5-Hydroxytryptophan - from Griffonia Bean) 50mg
- L-Theanine 50mg
- Hops Flower Extract 30mg
- Wild Lettuce Leaf Extract 22mg
- Lemon Balm Extract 20mg

I read about this product in Dr. Jacob Teitelbaum's book: *"From Fatigued to Fantastic: A Clinically Proven Program to Regain Vibrant Health and Overcome Chronic Fatigue and Fibromyalgia"*.

It's a good quality product and probably one of the strongest herbal remedies available for improving sleep, but despite all the ingredients supposedly proven to aid sleep, I unfortunately experienced no improvement, and didn't notice any effect whatsoever.

## Nutri MegaMag Night Formula powder

https://www.amazon.co.uk/MegaMag-Night-Formula-L-Tryptophan-L-Theanine/dp/B00YH3ICE2

These were recommended as one of the first things to try by a nutritionist. Despite trying this for 2-months, I unfortunately noticed no effect and no improvement in sleep.

The use of magnesium supplementation may be a prerequisite for moving onto adrenal glandular extracts and other supplements for helping to restore low-functioning adrenals. This is covered in a later section. But, suffice it to say, it is recommended that you seek guidance from a nutritionist before embarking on a course of supplementation.

## Yogi Soothing Caramel Bedtime Tea

https://www.amazon.co.uk/gp/product/B005OS39W4

I learnt about the Yogi Soothing Caramel Bedtime Tea in Timothy Ferriss' excellent book: *"Tools of Titans: The Tactics, Routines, and Habits of Billionaires, Icons, and World-Class Performers"*.

Ingredients:
- Organic California Poppy Plant 19mg
- L-Theanine Suntheanine 8mg
- Proprietary Blend of Herbs 1,738mg
    - Organic Chamomile Flower
    - Organic Rooibos Leaf
    - Organic Roasted Chicory Root
    - Organic Skullcap Leaf
    - Organic Nutmeg Kernal
    - Organic Cinnamon Bark

- Organic Stevia Leaf
- Organic Cardamon Pod
- Organic Ginger Root
- Organic Clove Bud
- Organic Black Pepper

I tried taking this tea around 9:30pm each evening and I did notice that it would help to make me even more sleepy than usual and is helpful with getting to sleep when first going to bed. I also like the flavour of the tea and have continued drinking it each evening. But, alas, it didn't seem to help with staying asleep throughout the night, but that's less of an issue nowadays anyway, as you'll read in later chapters.

**Nytol One-A-Night 50mg**
Advertised heavily on TV.
https://www.nytol.co.uk/nytol-range/
The active ingredient is diphenhydramine hydrochloride, an antihistamine that causes sleepiness or drowsiness. I tried Nytol a long while ago. It does help with falling asleep when first going to bed, but I would still wake in the night and didn't seem to get any extra sleep and felt a little more groggy than normal the next day so I stopped taking them.

They may have improved since I last took them, but I've avoided them since as I don't have a problem going to sleep but rather staying asleep.

It's also recommended to not take Nytol One-A-Night for more than 2 weeks without consulting your doctor. So you then have the issue of using them as a crutch for sleep and your body building up a tolerance for them, and then the issue of what happens when you stop taking them. And, as with the Sominex tablets, you also need to be careful not to take Nytol together with any other antihistamine tablets.

### Nytol Herbal Tablets
Zero improvement in sleep. No noticeable effect.

## Summary on Products, Pills and Remedies

Pretty much all the pills, products and herbal remedies listed above can be binned. They simply aren't needed to fix your sleep. I found that in the end, sorting out my dietary habits, daily routine and sleep hygiene (and sticking with it) was much more effective, which you'll soon read in about in the following chapters.

A cautionary note: it is not recommended to simply stop taking any current sleep medication, or any other medication (including natural remedies) without the advice of your doctor and/or nutritionist. But in the long run, based on my experience, you'll never be completely free from insomnia until you've stopped taking all sleeping medication.

Sleep is a natural process. There are millions of years of evolution behind the process of sleeping. Let's see if we can reclaim that natural cycle without the interference of drugs and other remedies.

# Chapter 3

## Other Methods I Tried

For completeness, in this chapter, I'd like to talk about other methods that I've tried over the years. Again, most of which, had little or no effect on the quality of my night time sleep, but I've added here for interest and because they may prove useful in some cases.

**Oral Device for Sleep Apnoea**

A sleep specialist I had several consultations with, at great expense, suggested I have a full blown sleep analysis conducted for one night. The sleep analysis was done at my own home with a representative coming to my house late in the evening to setup the device before I retired to bed. It wasn't exactly comfortable with the many wires and devices attached to me and I wasn't able to move around easily, so my sleep was even more disturbed than usual, but I was hopeful that some useful insights could be gleaned from the results. The same representative then returned to my house in the morning to collect up the sleep analysis device and all the wires so that the night's data could be analysed and collated.

The consultant thought that I might have a mild form of sleep apnoea based on the results of the sleep analysis. So I invested £1,500 getting a specialised oral device, custom made to fit tightly over my teeth and which moved my bottom jaw forward slightly to help ensure the airway stays open. It's like wearing a mouth guard, only it feels tighter over the teeth and slightly less comfortable.

I tried wearing the oral device for 2 weeks but really struggled to get on with it. I found it a little distracting and uncomfortable and it actually ended up keeping me awake longer. By 2am I'd give up and pry it out of my mouth. Later on I got a 2nd opinion on my sleep analysis results from another sleep and respiratory specialist and he saw no evidence of sleep apnoea. So that was a bust as well.

The oral device has helped many people that genuinely suffer with sleep apnoea, and may be more user-friendly than a cumbersome CPAP machine, but in my particular case it just wasn't needed. In hindsight I should have obtained a second opinion on my results before forking out for the custom-made oral device.

## CBT and Other Therapies

Cognitive Behavioral Therapy (CBT), along with maintaining good sleep hygiene, which the CBT courses promote and provide guidance on, all helped to improve my sleep a little. It didn't completely cure my broken sleep, but it did help move it in the right direction.

A Cognitive Behavioral Therapy course might be something your doctor advises as a first step, which is at least better than immediately writing a prescription.

**Sleepio**
https://www.sleepio.com/
Sleepio is an online Cognitive Behavioral Therapy (CBT) based program. I found this course to be very well put together and helped with regards to achieving and maintaining good sleep hygiene, which can be one of the biggest factors in gaining any improvements in sleep. However, at the time when I took the course, it seemed to focus more on getting to sleep rather than staying asleep. And in my particular case it didn't really resolve my sleep maintenance insomnia.

**The Sleep School**
https://thesleepschool.org/
The Sleep School is also an online Cognitive Behavioral Therapy (CBT) based program, similar to Sleepio but with more emphasis on negative thought processes and about staying in bed rather than getting up when you're awake in the night. This is also a good course and again helps with regards to achieving and maintaining good sleep hygiene. However, as with Sleepio, I was still not getting very good sleep. And as I mentioned in the introduction I just kind of failed at the whole 'just letting go' thing.

So I learnt a lot, but they didn't really solve my insomnia. I was still waking for long periods each night and was still feeling desperately weary every day.

It's easy to feel despondent having completed another course and not achieving any lasting benefits compared to the many positive reviews, especially when most of the pills and remedies also have little effect. You can really start to wonder what is actually wrong with you, which of course just adds to the challenges around sleep.

## Alternative Therapies and Products

### Paul McKenna's 'Sleep Like a Log' CD Audiobook
https://www.amazon.co.uk/Sleep-Like-Log-Paul-McKenna/dp/1900148110
This is quite an old product now, but all sound advice for helping to promote a good night's sleep. I listened to this in the daytime and would usually drift asleep within seconds of listening to it, which would essentially count as a daytime nap. I listened to this every day for many months, and despite it helping to relax me I didn't notice any improvements in the quality or quantity of my sleep, but I'd still say it's worth trying this. I also tried listening to this at night, when waking up and not being able to get back to sleep. I'd certainly feel relaxed, but alas, wouldn't actually fall asleep!

### HypSomnia E-Book and Audio File
https://twitter.com/hypsomnia
Similar to Paul McKenna's audio CD, this hypnotherapy CD would also cause me to get nicely relaxed and drift off to sleep in the daytime. But again, wouldn't get me back to sleep

when waking in the night. Maybe I should be a vampire - sleeping better in the daytime and being wide awake at night - right?

## Hypnotherapy

I tried three different courses of hypnotherapy with different therapists in my local area. The first sessions I tried, dates back to 2004. From the hypnotherapy sessions I had, it was interesting and quite disturbing to learn that my mind had apparently linked sleeping too long as being potentially life-threatening and was waking me up as a protection/survival instinct type thing. This was apparently triggered by some event dating way back to my early childhood. I don't know whether that's true or not, but it is one possible explanation as to why I stubbornly woke after only a few hours, and wasn't able to get back sleep. But despite the therapists' best efforts, I still found no improvements in my sleep, or any real change, and this included the use of personalised, hypnotherapy audio recordings that they'd provided for me to use between sessions.

I did find hypnotherapy to be very relaxing though, which is a definite plus point.

## Acupuncture

I tried two different courses of acupuncture treatment, with two different practitioners. Each course consisted of 10 separate sessions, conducted over a period of several weeks.

For me personally, I didn't notice any improvement in sleep, or, in fact, any effect whatsoever, and I didn't particularly enjoy the acupuncture as I'm not a great fan of needles. The practitioners were very careful and professional, but the treatment just didn't do anything and wasn't particularly comfortable for me.

**Binaural Beats - both with white noise and music**
https://www.youtube.com/results?search_query=binaural+beats+sleep
I tried having binaural beats sounds playing to aid sleep. I tried with headphones (see below AGPTEK headphones specially designed to wear while sleeping) and I tried without headphones. I tried listening to binaural beats with background white noise and binaural beats with music. I think it helped with relaxation but I personally didn't notice any improvements with sleep. I personally preferred the 'Deep White Noise with Binaural Beats for Sleep | Delta Waves Sleeping Sound | 10 Hours' track available on YouTube (https://www.youtube.com/watch?v=5V-oI-z1NgI). I had to keep my phone turned over and out the way on the floor so there was no light visible from the video... using the Griffin Bluetooth Wireless Adaptor (see below) was therefore useful.

On a related note, I have found a different type of binaural beats to be useful during the daytime when trying to concentrate on some work, especially when there's lots of noise around. I wear some noise-cancelling headphones and find the binaural beats concentration tracks to be helpful.

**AGPTEK Headband Headphones** with Lycra Mesh Lining and Carry Bag for Sleeping, Sports, Travel, Meditation

https://www.amazon.co.uk/gp/product/B074V5M18X
I found these headphones to be comfortable to wear while lying on my side in bed, which enabled me to still adopt my usual sleeping position while at the same time listening to an audio track (whether it's a hypnotherapy track or binaural beats track, etc.). I used these headphones in conjunction with Griffin Bluetooth Wireless Adaptor (see below) and my iPhone.

### Griffin Bluetooth Wireless Adaptor

https://www.amazon.co.uk/gp/product/B01HRYAP1K
This product is useful for allowing my iPhone to charge and be hidden out of the way, while at the same time playing audio without the need for long headphone cables etc. I could have the adaptor connected to the AGPTEK Headband Headphones and in a convenient place in the bed.

### Flux software

https://justgetflux.com/
This software is recommended to help reduce harmful blue light which can negatively impact on sleep and eye strain. I have it installed on my desktop and laptop and it works well. It hasn't magically fixed my sleep but I feel it helps to stack things in my favour for getting a better night's sleep.

### Blue Light Blocking Glasses

I've tried several different blue light blocking glasses, including Swanwick Blue Light Blocking Glasses (https://www.amazon.co.uk/gp/product/B010B5GUH0) which are one of the products recommended in Shawn

Stevenson's book "*Sleep Smarter: 21 Essential Strategies to Sleep Your Way to a Better Body, Better Health, and Bigger Success*".

Personally I didn't notice any improvements in my sleep as I think these are better suited to people suffering with sleep onset insomnia rather than sleep maintenance insomnia. Also I didn't particularly like the orange tint of the Swanwick Blue Light Blocking Glasses. It became slightly annoying when watching TV and using my computer and electronic devices to have the orange hue.

However I do recommend **DUCO Blue Light Blocking Glasses** (https://www.amazon.co.uk/gp/product/B00EJ4PTKE). I wear these whenever using my computer or iPad as I've found they help to prevent getting tired eyes and the eye strain from extended computer use, which is particularly noticeable when you're suffering with prolonged sleep deprivation and your eyes are already stinging before you even sit down in front of a screen.

**Philips HF3330 goLITE BLU Energy SAD Light**
https://www.amazon.co.uk/gp/product/B002G1Y8S6
I tried this product each day and evening for several weeks, but I didn't notice any effect on energy, mood, or any improvements in sleep at night. Apparently it is helpful for staying awake later into the evening, so you can better manage a more sensible sleep schedule in cases of sleep maintenance insomnia, i.e. where it is increasingly difficult to stay awake in the evening. However, for me I didn't notice any improvements in this area.

### Earthing

Earthing (reconnecting the human body to the Earth's surface electrons) was also something recommended in Shawn Stevenson's book "*Sleep Smarter: 21 Essential Strategies to Sleep Your Way to a Better Body, Better Health, and Bigger Success*". It's basically spending a short amount of time each day making barefoot contact with the earth's surface - usually just by walking or standing on grass or on the beach.

It's also possible to purchase an Earthing Sheet with Grounding Connection Cord which goes on your bed and allows you to be 'earthed' the entire time you're asleep (https://www.amazon.co.uk/Earthing-Grounding-Connection-Protection-60x80in/dp/B07S4MWRZL/). It's not a product I've tried personally, but looks promising for allowing more regular earthing sessions.

There have been numerous studies conducted on the health benefits of regular earthing. I tried this daily for about 10 minutes for numerous weeks, but didn't notice any improvement in sleep. However, I do think it helped a little with regards to more quickly over-coming jet lag when I was away on holiday. Just watch out for insect bites, which of course I got on my ankle the very first day I tried this!

### Meditation

From what I've read on this, I think meditation could be a real benefit and help to improve the problems of getting back to sleep after waking. I've tried meditating on many occasions, at different times of the day, however the challenge I faced here was that I almost immediately nodded off to sleep once closing my eyes and getting into a relaxed state, and then my head would lull forward and I'd jerk back awake. This micro sleep and sudden jerking awake would happen several times and would almost always result in a headache.

So for me, it seems like a chicken-and-egg situation where I'd need to have a reasonable amount of sleep so I'm not too sleepy to be able to meditate, but I'd need to meditate so I was able to get a reasonable amount of sleep.

A friend suggested I try a rocking-back-and-forth type of meditation in order to stay awake, but I wasn't sure I could stomach the repetitive rocking with my eyes closed. And, in fact, another friend of hers tried this rocking-back-and-forth type of meditation and did eventually spew, so yeah I'm steering clear of that method.

I have found mindful breathing mediation to be helpful when lying awake at night. I'll talk more on this in a later chapter, but you simply lie on your back in a relaxed comfortable position, eyes closed, and gently bring your attention to your breathing. Focus your attention on the gentle rise and fall of the abdomen or the air flowing in and out of your nose. If the mind gets distracted by other thoughts, just notice that and again gently return your focus back to your breathing.

## OOLER® Sleep System

https://www.chilitechnology.com/products/ooler-sleep-system

The OOLER® Sleep System is an advanced sleep system for controlling the temperature of your bed. It comes with a hydronic pad and control unit and can be controlled via an app. The hydronic pad is a mattress topper which incorporates thin circulation tubes. Water is circulated from the control unit through the tubes and efficiently maintains a consistent temperature.

It's quite expensive, but is brilliant for helping to maintain a consistent body temperature throughout the night and thereby helping to prevent waking in the night from being too hot.

## Exerpeutic 475SL Inversion Table

https://www.amazon.co.uk/gp/product/B07B28WKX8

An inversion table allows you to gently and comfortably tilt yourself into a 180 degree vertical inversion while being held securely via the ankles. It's supposed to do wonders for your back by decompressing your spine, and people have reported that this also helps improve sleep.

I learnt about the use of inversion tables in Timothy Ferriss' book: *"Tools of Titans: The Tactics, Routines, and Habits of Billionaires, Icons, and World-Class Performers"*.

There are many different types of inversion tables available. I opted for the Exerpeutic 475SL. It's pretty heavy and required two-person assembly from the flat-pack. It also requires quite a lot of space to be used, as you rotating over in a circular type motion. But it does fold away allowing slightly easier storage.

It took a little getting used to and is definitely worth taking it slowly to start with. You simply raise your arms slowly and gradually up over your head and the table effortless tilts on its fulcrum. Tilt back a little to start with and then slowly return back to the upright position, gradually you can increase the angle as you feel more comfortable, but you should always tilt back gradually both when going back and when returning to the upright position.

To achieve the full 180 degree vertical inversion you have to reach your arms fully over your head and use the supporting bar at the bottom of the A-frame to gently increase yourself to the full 180 degrees.

Now that I'm used to it I actually enjoy it and find it relaxing, and I have already noticed that it has helped ease lower back pain I tend to experience.

However on the downside it hasn't had any noticeable effect on my sleep and really does need a lot of space.

## Other References

If you're interested in keeping up to date with the latest sleep related gadgets then I can recommend checking out the sleepgadgets.io website. It provides independent, expert reviews, and showcases sleep gadgets and circadian health technology including bestsellers on Amazon, and crowdfunding innovations on Kickstarter and IndieGogo.

I can also recommend the sleepjunkies.com website as a good source of all the latest information on sleep. They publish a range of content covering every aspect of sleep, from blog posts to interviews, feature articles, product reviews, and news.

However, just a cautionary note here... focusing too heavily on all the latest sleep related news and relying on too many gadgets can backfire and add to the anxiety around sleep.

# Chapter 4

## Napping and Coping with Broken Sleep

Napping is a double-edged sword. It might help to relieve the chronic tiredness for short periods, but it does ultimately affect the quality of sleep at night, especially for those suffering with long term sleep problems.

I got to the point where I was so addicted to napping, it felt like I couldn't survive without at least 2 or 3 naps per day. I was so used to getting very short bursts of sleep, this became the norm, even when going to bed at night. I'd lie down to sleep and it would feel like I'd immediately plunge into a deep sleep, only to snap back out of it after a few minutes, then be wide awake. I was stuck in a cycle of just getting these very short bursts of sleep. Deep down, I knew I had to break the cycle of napping.

This is one area that bugs me about other sleep books, and guidance given during therapy sessions. They all basically say you shouldn't nap during the day, which is all very sound advice. They just don't give any practical guidance on how to *avoid* napping. It seems simple enough, right... just don't nap during the day. Hmm, yeah, well for me it was like going cold turkey from some kind of drug addiction. It would be like asking a 60-a-day cigarette smoker to simply stop smoking, and that being the end of the discussion. I feel like there should be some kind of nap-aholics anonymous support group or something!

There's also a lot of guidance out there on sleep restriction as a way to resolve broken sleep. I tried that as well, but it would either be torturous trying to stay awake so late into the night before sleeping, or I'd break through the extreme tiredness and end up getting some kind of second wind and then be awake for longer than I wanted, or I would usually just wake up long before the designated awake time anyway. So sleep restriction didn't really work for me. It just seemed overly harsh when you're already desperately short of sleep.

But in fact, not napping during the day is one of the key components in breaking the cycle and helping to improve the quality of sleep – this also includes weekends. I know it's very tempting when you've been out of bed since 5am and probably awake for what seems like ages before that. The kids are out at football practice with your partner, or whatever, and you have some free time to kill. And all you want to do is lie down and die, and having that nap (sometimes an extended nap) can feel like the only way of getting through the day, and possibly even the highlight of the day when you're feeling so lousy. Believe me, I know. I know the desire to nap can be overwhelming sometimes. But unfortunately, from my long years of experience, it is really an important and necessary component in breaking out of the cycle and making real progress on fixing chronic insomnia. The pills and latest remedies aren't going to do it, not in the long run at least, not if your sleep has been broken for so long.

Imagine that insidious, malevolent dragon egging you on to sleep and rubbing its hands with glee, thinking "go on, do it, just have that nap, and I'll soon have this sucker back on the treadmill of insomnia"! You've got to resist the urge to nap in the daytime to break out of the cycle. I know it's tough at first, but it does get easier once you get over the initial few days and the quality of your night time sleep starts to improve.

I had some particularly tricky times when I was trying to stop napping while simultaneously stopping sleep medication and caffeine and reducing sugar intake. It was a recipe for a whole world of fun and games, and by fun and games I mean a tailspin of misery and despair. But you've got to be strong on this one, and stick with the routine and changes, and before too long you'll start feeling the benefits, and the quality of your sleep will improve. Hopefully you won't also have to simultaneously stop sleep medication, but it can still be tough at first.

Instead of napping, it would be far better to get your walking boots on and go out for a walk. Or do some gentle exercise at home if the weather is too unpleasant. Try to stay active that day and make it through to bedtime. It's worth it in the long run.

Just a cautionary note here though, because you do need to be careful when cutting out naps. Sometimes I felt very sleepy during long drives, and would have no choice but to pull over at the next service station for a short nap – usually to be woken by a door slamming nearby. Nevertheless, it was enough of a pick-me-up to be able drive safely again. This, of course, counted as a nap, but it's not worth the risk to drive while feeling too tired and sleepy. So you may want to plan ahead and start your no-napping sleep-reset program at a time when you don't have any long car journeys planned, especially at times when you're likely to be at your most sleepy during the day.

There will also be other obstacles that crop up along the way. For example, I fell ill with appendicitis and had to have two short stays in hospital. This was right at the time when I was going through the weeks of breaking the cycle of napping. It seemed like slightly suspicious timing and very convenient for the curse of insomnia. The timing is probably just a coincidence, but I can't help wondering if it had anything to do with all the chopping and changing with different sleep medications and herbal remedies I'd tried. Unfortunately, hospitals are not the best place for maintaining optimal sleep hygiene. They're quite noisy and light throughout the night, and you're in bed all day, you're not getting any exercise and are likely to drift off to sleep when you shouldn't be. So I did get better from the illness, but the stay in hospital basically reset my progress, and I had to start my routine all over again.

So, what did I do to break the cycle of napping? Initially, I limited myself to having no more than 1 nap per day, and for no more than 15 minutes, and definitely not after 3pm. I stuck with that rule for a while, including making sure I had a nap before any long afternoon drives if I felt I needed one. And then after a few days, I bit-the-bullet and cut out napping altogether.

Sometimes I felt so sleepy during the day that I'd have to try various things to stop myself nodding off. I'd have a shower and gradually turn the water to run cold for a while before getting out, or I'd just simply splash some cold water onto my face. I'd go out for a walk. I'd put some music on and play dancing games with my kids. I'd do some stretching exercises. Deep breathing exercises. Clean out a cupboard, or a room. Do some cooking. Listen to music - particularly music from your youth, or any energising or uplifting music (such as "Eye of the Tiger" by Survivor, or "Don't Stop Me Now" by Queen, or "Move Your Body" by Sia). Or I'd play chasing games with my kids, basically anything to stay more active and alert to help stop myself from nodding off. Just sitting and watching TV, or reading, or studying, or playing/browsing on my iPad, or doing something sedentary and boring was a no-no at those times of increased sleepiness. After a little while, the feelings of sleepiness would lift enough to keep me going until bed time.

And in terms of trying to stay awake and as alert as possible throughout the work day, it's helpful, if at all possible, to try to prioritise work you can get actively engaged in. I'm not just talking about physically active. I also mean mentally engaging, especially aspects of your work that you enjoy and where you lose track of time. Ideally, where you're able to completely forget about time and get into a state of 'flow'. You won't feel tired and time will seem to pass much more quickly. For me, this is programming. I try to work on projects that I can get most absorbed in.

To learn more about this concept of 'flow' and about the work that is actively engaging for you then I recommend checking out the books *'The Element: How Finding Your Passion Changes Everything'* and *'Finding Your Element: How to Discover Your Talents and Passions and Transform Your Life'* by Sir Ken Robinson.

If you're sat in boring meetings all day, even the best of sleepers will feel like snoozing. But you may be limited in what's possible, depending on your occupation and work and responsibilities, etc. The more active and/or the more you're engaged in work, or past time activities you find stimulating, the better for being able to stay awake and alert throughout the day.

What can also be a challenge is that you won't necessarily see immediate improvements to the quality of your sleep, especially if your sleep has been broken for a long time. It takes time for your body to gradually and naturally correct its circadian rhythm, so you've got to stick with it before the gains start to appear. Unfortunately, it seems to be the case that the longer you've had broken sleep the longer it takes to fix. It's like you get through one day of not napping, only to have another bad night, and you think "you've got to be kidding me." This was another reason why making the other changes and having much improved energy levels – which I'll talk about in detail – was so beneficial for me, because it really helped me to have the strength to persevere through the initial dip in the road. If I was still feeling lethargic with poor energy levels as a results of years of poor dietary habits, then trying to stick with the strict sleep hygiene becomes all that more difficult. All this will be covered soon.

Once the quality of your sleep improves and your energy levels are more stable, then you won't need to jump through all the hoops trying to stay awake. I gradually found I was naturally more active and more alert. The brain fog had lifted too. And I didn't have such trouble staying awake throughout the day, which all in turn led to better quality sleep each night. I could finally start to feel the benefits and get off the vicious downward cycle, and instead get onto the virtuous cycle.

Just one thing to mention about sleep apnoea and how it relates to daytime napping, which I know I said I wasn't going to cover in this book, but this is a fairly important point to include in this chapter. If you have sleep apnoea, then it's unlikely you'll be able to stop daytime napping. If you find it is almost impossible to stop yourself from nodding off in the daytime, then there's a good chance you have sleep apnoea, and it is therefore highly advisable to get a referral from your doctor to have that treated as soon as possible. You'll most likely be asked to complete an Epworth Sleepiness Scale, which is used to diagnose obstructive sleep apnoea. It's a questionnaire used to help determine how likely you are to fall asleep in various situations, in comparison to feeling tired.

For example: https://www.blf.org.uk/support-for-you/obstructive-sleep-apnoea-osa/diagnosis/epworth-sleepiness-scale

# The Effects of Napping

One downside you might initially face when forcing yourself not to nap is that it can paradoxically end up putting more pressure on going to sleep when you're finally 'allowed' to go to bed. And that pressure can end up pushing sleep away because you start feeling tense and worried because sleeping at night has become even more important. I've very rarely had that problem. I'm usually so tired by night time, I'm in danger of falling asleep while brushing my teeth. People with sleep maintenance insomnia don't usually have problems going to sleep, but if you feel the anxiety start to creep in, then it's advisable to get more relaxed in the evening before going to bed. For example, I'd recommend watching funny movies and TV shows rather than heart-thumping, high energy movies. For example, choose Monty Python's Life of Brian over the latest horror movie. Or read a relaxing book, preferably not on an electronic device. Or have a bath with your preferred bath salts added.

And don't be tempted to go to bed too early. As well as not napping, it's also important to stick with regular bedtimes and regular times when you're out of bed in the morning. These of course need to be sensible levels and should be the same at weekends as well as week days. An example might be going to bed at 11pm and getting out of bed at 6pm. That's 7 hours of possible sleep time. If you find yourself lucky enough to start easily sleeping through that time then you can adjust either the time of going to bed, or the time of getting out of bed.

In Dr. James L. Wilson's book '*Adrenal Fatigue: The 21st Century Stress Syndrome*', he recommends:

> *"For people with adrenal fatigue (most people), it is important to be in bed and asleep before your second wind hits at about 11:00 PM. Riding your second wind and staying up until 1:00 or 2:00 in the morning will further exhaust your adrenals, even though you may feel more energetic during that time than you have felt all day. In order to avoid this pitfall, make sure that you are in bed and on your way to sleep before 10:30 PM, so that your adrenal glands do not have a chance to kick into overdrive for that second wind.*

> *"Although most people's schedules do not allow it, it also helps to sleep in until 8:30 or 9:00. There is something magical about the restorative power of sleep between 7:00-9:00 in the morning for people with adrenal fatigue. Even when your night has been restless or your sleep fitfull, catching those couple of hours of sleep between 7:00-9:00 AM can be remarkably refreshing."* (124)

I struggle to stay awake past 10:30pm anyway, so I tend to go with his first point as being a good time to go to bed. Sleeping between 7:00 to 9:00am is little more tricky when you're trying to resolve chronic sleep maintenance insomnia. I've tried this on rare occasions when it's been possible and, yes it was delicious sleep and certainly helped relieve the feelings of sleepiness for a short while in the day, but for me it just seemed to affect the quality of sleep that night and therefore perpetuated the broken sleep. And of course I could only try this on rare occasions when I didn't have other day time responsibilities that needed attention. I found I simply had to stick with the no sleeping in the daytime routine to give my night time sleep chance to stabilise and fully restore.

I tried to quantify the effects of daytime napping on night time sleep, which was of course almost impossible to quantify because there are so many other variables that can affect sleep, and my sleep was erratic at the best of times, but as a rough guide, based on my own experimentations and patterns of insomnia, I reckoned that about 20 minutes of day time sleep would equate to about 1 hour of lost sleep at night. That's how sensitive my night time sleep had become over the years and why I had to break the cycle to have any chance of resolve the quality of my night time sleep.

Once your sleep is in a much better place and you've been sleeping well consistently for many months, it might be okay to re-introduce short naps at appropriate times. Probably a normal sleeper wouldn't think twice about having a nice nap when possible. Personally I wouldn't want to risk breaking the much improved sleep/wake cycle, but that's really because my sleep was broken for so long. Better to let the improved patterns of sleep become much more established before slipping back to old habits.

# Products to Help Manage Headaches

I've included this section here for all those that currently suffer with recurring headaches.

I used to have headaches almost on a daily basis especially after a particularly bad night. So I've tried a number of different products over the years to help deal with the seemingly never-ending stream of headaches.

Nowadays, since making the changes described later in this book and because I'm sleeping a whole lot better, I thankfully hardly ever get headaches, which is just one of the many huge benefits of the changes and improved sleep.

But if you do currently suffer with headaches while on the road to much improved sleep, then the list below may be helpful.

### White Tiger Balm Ointment
https://www.amazon.co.uk/gp/product/B002QQN37S
I was sceptical that a balm could stop a headache, but to my surprise and delight I found Tiger Balm to be a brilliant little product at relieving mild headaches. Often times I can apply Tiger Balm when I feel a headache coming on and it will actually stop a headache in its tracks and prevent the need for taking any medication. This is particularly useful for me as the headaches would often occur in the evening and the only medication that would seem to work for me contains caffeine (see below) and therefore is detrimental to sleep.

**Anadin Extra**

https://www.anadin.co.uk/our-products/anadin-extra-anadin-extra-soluble

These tablets usually help to get rid of headaches for me. The tablets contain aspirin (300mg), paracetamol (200mg) and caffeine (45mg). Interestingly, I've tried just taking aspirin and it doesn't seem to get rid of my headaches. I've tried just taking paracetamol and that also doesn't seem to get rid of my headaches. I've also tried taking both aspirin and paracetamol and that too doesn't seem to get rid of my headaches. Rather annoyingly it seems the addition of caffeine is required before the headaches are quashed. And the caffeine can of course negatively impact sleep. However if it's a choice between lying awake with a headache or lying awake without a headache, then I'll choose the latter and take the tablets particularly if it's a bad headache.

But these tablets should really be an absolute last resort, reserved for particularly bad headaches only, because the caffeine is really not helpful while you're on the road to fixing your sleep.

As an alternative you could try a much stronger dose of paracetamol, for example most pharmacies and supermarkets stock 500mg tablets with the recommended dosage being 2 tablets every 6 hours. So it's likely that a 1000mg dose of paracetamol will be enough for most headaches and has saved the need for taking a tablet containing caffeine.

Obviously you can't then take another tablet also containing paracetamol within that 6 hour window otherwise you risk an overdose.

## Alka-Seltzer XS

https://www.amazon.co.uk/Alka-Seltzer-XS-Effervescent-Tablets/dp/B000KU51ZO/

I have noticed that the Anadin Extra tablets described above seem to be regularly out of stock, at least in my local area. So the Alka-Seltzer XS tablets could be used as an alternative. They also contain aspirin (267mg per tablet), paracetamol (133mg per tablet) and caffeine (40mg per tablet), and seem to be more readily available. They work just as well as Anadin Extra and also dissolve more quickly compared to the soluble version of Anadin Extra.

## Natures Aid Ucalm St John's Wort Extract, 300 mg, 60 Tablets

https://www.amazon.co.uk/gp/product/B0074I668G

These herbal tablets are marketed as a relief from the symptoms of slightly low mood and mild anxiety. I personally didn't notice any effect when taking these.

## Neobun Menthol Plaster

https://www.amazon.co.uk/Neobun-Menthol-Plaster-Sheets-Relieve/dp/B00BM6L82K

As with the Tiger Balm, I was sceptical that a plaster applied to the skin would stop a headache, but again these menthol plasters seemed to work in some instances and are usually sufficient to get rid of mild headaches, which again prevent the need for taking the caffeine based medication.

The only slight downside is that you have to walk around with a large patch stuck to your forehead or temples, so popping to the shops might raise some strange looks.

**HeadaTerm TENS Device - Electrode Stimulator for Headache Relief**
https://www.amazon.co.uk/gp/product/B072JSSR95
Interesting product, but sadly for me personally it didn't help to get rid of my headaches.

# Chapter 5

## The Foundations

Okay. Now that we've dealt with all the negative stuff, let's get down to what really worked for me. I'm going to say, right off the bat that fixing my sleep wasn't easy. That's why this book is called The Long Road to Sleep. It wasn't a quick pit stop at the pharmacy and bang you're done. There wasn't a miracle cure, or sudden breakthrough. It took some dogged persistence and there were some setbacks along the way. So I'm sorry to disappoint if you're looking for that one quick fix, that one magic pill, the silver-bullet. For me at least, it took months and a lot of self-navigation through the maze of solutions, a lot of trial and error before I found what worked. With the benefit of hindsight, I could have saved myself a lot of trouble and fixed my sleep within about 4 weeks. I say 4 weeks because even knowing what finally worked for me, it still took a lot of time to break the 30+ years of broken sleep.

So you're going to get the benefit of my hindsight and depending on how long you've been suffering with insomnia you could even fix your sleep in a much shorter time. But please be prepared for sticking with things for weeks rather than days before you start to get the benefits. Keep the goal of improved sleep in mind and don't give up. As I mentioned, it does seems to be the case that the longer you've had broken sleep, the longer it takes to fix. But it is possible to fix, so keep that in mind.

Before we begin on the changes needed to fix decades of insomnia, we need to ensure we're set up for enabling the best possible sleep. Uh oh, I'm going to drone on about sleep hygiene now aren't I? Don't worry I'll save you the bother of reading chapter and verse on sleep hygiene. I'm sure you're already an expert if you've been suffering with chronic insomnia for many years. I'm just going to list here the things I have in place to help ensure I have the best possible night sleep. Sticking with a good routine and maintaining impeccable sleep hygiene is important for fixing decades of broken sleep. Each item I've listed on its own isn't going to magically fix your sleep, but you want to give yourself the best possible chance of a great night's sleep in the best possible environment, so that when you start on the other changes it can all come together nicely.

**Mattress**: Fairly obvious one here, but you want to have the most comfortable bed you can find for yourself. I tried many mattresses over the years and have found the Simba Hybrid Mattress is a good quality mattress at a reasonable price. It's firm without being too hard and comfortable without being too soft. I've used it for a few years now and it is still firm without showing hardly any signs of sagging. The Simba

customer services are very good too.
https://simbasleep.com/products/mattress

The only downside I noticed with the Simba mattress, which is true for many other mattresses too, is that it can soak up and hold onto body heat. The OOLER® Sleep System mentioned in the previous chapter can really help with this problem.

If you have the budget for it, I can recommend The Marriott Mattress as being one of the best mattresses available.
https://europe.shopmarriott.com/en/marriott-mattress
Superb quality and comfort and it doesn't soak up body heat quite so much.

**Pillow**: Simba Hybrid® Pillow with OUTLAST®
https://simbasleep.com/products/simba-hybrid-pillow
There are so many different types of pillows available, made with all manner of different materials and all manner of shapes and sizes that it can be a bit bewildering trying to choose what might be the most comfortable. Also each person seems to have a different preferred favourite. In our household alone my son swears by the Sweet Dreams contoured memory foam pillow, whereas my girlfriend prefers a completely different natural fibre pillow.

I've tried various different pillows and have found my personal favourite is the Simba Hybrid® Pillow. I personally prefer the side of the pillow with the OUTLAST® material, which apparently was originally developed for space exploration, and proactively regulates your body temperature by absorbing, storing and releasing heat. And the side gusset on the pillow is helpful as I sleep on my side so need a little extra support in the pillow.

The Simba pillow arrives crammed quite full of the foam Nanocubes, but you can remove them for the perfect height and firmness. The foam Nanocubes you don't need can be stored in a pouch provided and then added later on should you wish to increase the firmness.

It's also relatively easy to wash the cover as it simply unzips on one side and the inner pillow can be removed.

**Curtains**: I already had blackout lined curtains fitted, but there was still a small ingress of light around the top and side edges. So I also had a roller blind fitted snugly in the recess to sit behind the curtains. This pretty much blocks out all light and my room is pitch black at night time, which I've learnt is important for helping to improve sleep.

**Routine**: The time you go to bed and the time you get out of bed should be roughly the same every day, including on weekends and holidays. I've never ever needed an alarm clock, as is often the case for anyone suffering from sleep maintenance insomnia. I'd always be wide awake in the early hours way before I needed to be up. But regardless of this, I did structure a regular time of going bed, and I stuck with that, regardless of how the previous night was. I'd start going upstairs and getting ready for bed at around 10:00pm and have lights out around 10:30pm. And then I'm up at around 5:30 to 6:00am. I'll talk more about routine in a later chapter.

**Earplugs**: My sleep is easily disturbed by noise, so earplugs were helpful for me particularly when going back to sleep in the early hours of the morning when my sleep was lighter and the first sounds of the day would start in earnest. I just use the simple foam earplugs available in most supermarkets and pharmacies.

**Sleeping alone**: this is potentially a hot topic, but just to let you know what I did: my girlfriend is very supportive and agreed to let me sleep alone. This decision may have been helped due to her also being woken up regularly by my moving around and getting out of bed several times per night. We are planning to once again sleep in the same bed now that my sleep is much better.

**Napping**: another potentially worrying subject for chronic insomniacs is the temptation of napping. This was a problem and a challenge for me, as we covered in detail in the previous chapter. As we covered, try not to nap. It can only ruin the quality of your night time sleep rhythm.

**Caffeine**: Cut out caffeine after 1pm, preferably all together while going through the process of re-establishing a much improved circadian rhythm. Caffeine has quite a long half-life and stays in the system for many hours and can disrupt the delicate process maintaining the sleep-wake cycle. It is best avoided all together if you've been suffering with broken sleep for many years. You need to give your body chance to be stimulant-free and to reset the circadian rhythm.

Once your sleep is at a much better and more stable level then I think it's fine to have a relatively small amount of caffeine each day, for example 1 or 2 coffees or teas each morning, especially if you enjoy a nice hot beverage each morning. You shouldn't feel like you need to miss out on this. But it's best to completely avoid consuming caffeine after 3pm.

It's also best to avoid the energy drinks with high levels of caffeine as these are likely to play havoc with regards to maintaining stable energy levels throughout the day and are likely to impact on your sleep.

Just to give you some idea of the varying amounts of caffeine in the many different products available: A cup of Maxwell House Regular Ground Coffee has about 45-100mg of caffeine. A cup of green tea has about 28-38mg. A Starbucks caffe latte or cappucino has about 150mg. A Diet Coke has 46mg. Some of the heavy-hitters such as the Bang Energy drink has 300mg. And the Dunkin' Donuts coffee with espresso shot has about 398mg. And one 40g box of Crackheads Gourmet Chocolate Coffee Caffeine weighs in at a massive 600mg of caffeine!

Once you go beyond 400mg of caffeine per day you really start to enter overdose territory and are at risk of experiencing the unpleasant side-effects including dizziness, irregular heartbeat and seizures.

**Alcohol:** I can't really comment much on this as I don't drink alcohol, so this wasn't a possible issue for me. But every book states that alcohol can negatively impact on the body's natural sleep cycles and it is recommended that insomnia sufferers cut down or eliminate alcohol consumption in order to have the best chance of fixing broken sleep. It's certainly true that friends of mine, who either stopped drinking completely, or gave themselves a two-month break, all reported much better sleep.

Also, as you'll learn in a later chapter, alcohol has a highly acidifying affect in the body, it destroys cells, it interrupts everything and it overwhelms the body. If you want to give yourself the best chance of resolving your broken sleep it is highly recommended to cut down or completely cut out the consumption of alcohol.

**Antihistamines**: Antihistamines can cause sleepiness, including the non-drowsy variety, and from what I've read they can interfere with the body's natural circadian rhythm. I used to take an Antihistamine every morning for hay fever relief, however I initially changed to taking them every evening instead of in the morning. But I discovered that ultimately I no longer needed to take them due to the dietary changes I made, specifically cutting out foods I have an intolerance to. I'll talk a little more about this in a later chapter, but it's advisable to review your allergy medication to look at what and when you take them.

As with other medication, please consult with your doctor before changing the dosage or if you want to stop taking them.

**Phones and Electronic Devices:** This is such an obvious one, I nearly forgot to include it, but make sure your mobile phones, tablets, laptops and other such electronic devices are switched off, or at least switched to silent mode before going to bed. And with the screens facing down and away from the bed to ensure your sleep isn't disturbed by the sounds and lights from notifications. It's highly advisable not to look at your phone if you wake in the night. The light from the screen and possible notifications will only wake you up further.

**Clocks:** As well as not looking at your phone if you wake in the night, it is also advisable not to clock watch. However if you have a need to see what the time is in the night then I recommend using a clock that has a fully adjustable dimmer and have it set to the minimum possible level where you can only just see the numbers in total darkness, for example I use the Reacher LED Digital Alarm Clock with Full Range Brightness Dimmer:
https://www.amazon.co.uk/Reacher-Digital-Bedside-Operation-Brightness/dp/B07BKVVGDJ

**Also worth considering**: electriQ Compact 9000 BTU Small and Powerful Portable Air Conditioner
https://www.appliancesdirect.co.uk/p/compact/electriq-compact
I purchased this free-standing air-conditioning unit to use during the summer months. It was particularly useful during the run of hot weather we had last year. Despite the unit being quite loud and heavy I found it was a real god send during the heat wave and I ended up using it for about 8

weeks straight. My bedroom would have been much too hot to have any chance of a reasonable amount of sleep, so having the air-conditioning unit helped to get the room cool and comfortable.

If you wake up in the night feeling hot and have to kick the duvet off (or partially off) then your room is probably a little too hot. You ideally want to be aiming for cool but comfortable. In the winter months I have the radiator set on a fairly low level.

## Summary

I highly recommend getting your sleep environment and sleep hygiene into the best possible shape you can. If you've been suffering from years of insomnia, then you probably already know a lot about sleep hygiene.

This is your foundation, your bedrock to having the best chance of fixing broken sleep. So step 1 is to get your sleep environment and sleep hygiene sorted. You need bullet-proof sleep hygiene before you can get your broken sleep fixed for good. Think of it as the armour you need to fight off that fire-breathing dragon. Make your sleep hygiene solid and it will serve you well, but you need patience to realise the full benefits - 1 day of good sleep hygiene isn't going to immediately cure decades of insomnia.

# Chapter 6

## Energy - The Turning Point

Just take a step back for a moment and think about the bigger picture, think about why you're desperately trying to improve your sleep? It seems like an obvious question, right? I mean, why on earth would you not want to fix your sleep? If you're anything like me, your answers are probably something like: because you don't want to feel so lousy, or feel like the walking dead every day, or because you want to have the energy to do the things you want to do in your life, or because you're worried about ill-health and the negative effects of prolonged sleep deprivation, or because you're so tired of feeling tired all the time. Sound familiar?

For years I blamed my continual lack of energy all on sleep. I thought if I could just fix my sleep, everything would be ok, which in turn put more pressure on the need to sleep well, and more worry and more anxiety, which just made sleep even more difficult.

As this vicious cycle had been going on for so long, I really started to worry that my entire life was going to be lived running only on fumes. Never feeling energised and just generally not having the energy to do all the things I wanted to. Gradually, the worry, frustration and anxiety turned to despair. And that despair and desperation led me to trying anything I could get my hands on, sometimes with professional guidance, but usually by self-navigating through a forest of information and a huge range of pills, remedies, products and therapies as you've seen in previous chapters.

It also didn't help that the lethargy and continual lack of energy made it difficult to stick to a rock solid routine, and bullet-proof sleep hygiene, which in turn all compounded to make sleep even more broken, and further from my grasp.

It wasn't until I took a step back and started focusing on my lack of energy that things started to change. I didn't completely ignore my broken sleep - kind of hard to ignore that – but I had almost given up trying to fix it and switched my attention to my lack of energy which led to my first glimmer of hope. I thought maybe I could do something about this, regardless of my lack of sleep. So I began trying things to help improve my energy. At first I continued to make the mistake of trying various supplements and remedies, without any other changes or advice, which didn't help much. It wasn't until I found the dietary and lifestyle changes that things started to change for the better.

Let me repeat this important point – I stopped trying to fix my sleep, and instead worked on improving my energy. Sleep could go stand in the naughty corner for a while. I'm now playing with its younger sibling, energy! Giving energy my attention turned out to be the key that finally broke the vicious cycle.

And the other thing I noticed was that exercising daily became easier. But more to the point, I didn't need any kind of massive gruelling effort where you have to force yourself to get off the sofa to do some exercise. Instead it came with surprising ease. In fact, I really missed it if some event or reason caused me to skip my usual exercise schedule.

All of this then became a virtuous cycle. Feeling better, having more energy, exercising regularly, being more active and sticking with good sleep hygiene, finally started to resolve my decades of broken sleep. To my astonishment, I realised that I'd stopped worrying about sleep. That didn't mean I'd solved the problem; I just wasn't worrying about it.

This really is worth re-iterating: because I was feeling so much better each day, I really didn't worry so much about my sleep. I still suffered from lack of sleep, but it became less of an issue. And of course with all that pressure and worry finally out of the way, and with a much-improved routine, my sleep began to resolve itself.

Another way to think about this is, if you do manage to fix your sleep, but still feel like crap every day and have very low energy, then it's only half the job done – in my opinion. You want the whole package, right? You want to sleep well and feel good. So I found that it's important to work on your energy levels as well as your sleep. Or better yet, work on your energy levels and health, while maintaining a good routine and let sleep take care of itself.

So let's think about this. It's entirely possible to sleep well, but still feel rough. If poor health continues, it's possible to get to a point where the body demands more and more rest, and in some extreme cases could be almost entirely bedridden. Sleep might be increasing, but the quality of life gradually disappears as health declines. So it's important to not only take charge of the quality of your sleep, but also take charge of the quality of your health. It's more of a holistic approach, with the two going hand in hand.

What I finally discovered was that it's also possible to sleep only 6 hours, but still feel great. Gradually, your natural level of sleep – that's right for your body, because we're all different – will start to appear. It's all about setting up the right conditions to allow it to happen.

So the big turning point for me came when I shifted my focus to improving my lack of energy. It's a subtle change in attention, but it did several things. It took away a lot of the focus purely from sleep, and I did actually find things which significantly improved my energy. Having improved energy meant I was more active in the day and was better able to stick with my sleep improvement routines, which all in turn led to fixing my sleep.

This shift in attention onto fixing my lack of energy took me on another quest of finding answers that actually worked, and this is what this part of the book is all about. I looked into Chronic Fatigue Syndrome, Fibromyalgia and Adrenal Fatigue. And as when trying to fix my sleep, I tried a range of different supplements, dietary and lifestyle changes and read numerous books. Many things had little or no impact, but eventually I found some things that really worked for me.

Just a note here in terms of focus and attention... I'm not talking about the silly mind games, which seem so prevalent in many other books and courses, where you just have to 'let go' of worrying about insomnia and that it's not that a big of deal. Every book seems to say the same thing about just letting go. Yeah, right. I don't know about you, but I completely failed at just trying to ignore it and letting go. It felt like I was just trying to fool myself and ignore the elephant in the room, I'm sorry, but decades of insomnia is a bloody big deal, thank you very much! However, I did find that shifting my attention to fixing my debilitating lack of energy helped to take a lot of the pressure off it all being about sleep.

I also discovered that it's possible to have a lot more energy even after only 6 hours sleep? 6 hours! But I'm only getting a fraction of that. Yep, I hear you. So sleep is still the primary focus of this book. Just have an open mind that improving your energy leads to improving sleep. It's like a virtuous cycle and it's a long road. One step at a time. Well actually, we can do a few steps at a time, but I'll get to that.

Ok I'm sold, how do I fix my energy problems? As with sleep, I went through a raft of books, products, herbal remedies and various dietary changes while on the quest to improve my energy levels. And once again, most didn't help. But the following items had the most positive impact for me, not only in improving and stabilising my energy levels but also improving my overall health:

Which brings me onto the work of Dr Alex Guerrero and his book *In Balance for Life: Understanding and Maximizing Your Body's pH Factor*. Dr Alex Guerrero is an alternative medicine practitioner, who is best known as an advocate of the alkaline based diet and for his work with professional American football players. What's interesting is that Dr Guerrero can not only turn around peak performance athletes when they're burning out, but he also specializes in taking care of patients that traditional doctors think are terminal and inoperable. He's now cared for 400 terminal patients designated as untreatable by their physicians. Several years later approximately 85% of them are still alive and thriving.

Dr Guerrero is also recommended by Tony Robbins in the 'Pure Energy Live' seminar section of his '*Get the Edge*' audio program. Specifically Disc 6 (Day 4) of the program, which covers in detail how to significantly improve your energy and is based on the work of Dr Alex Guerrero.

I highly recommend checking out Tony Robbins' '*Get the Edge*' audio program and Dr Alex Guerrero book *In Balance for Life: Understanding and Maximizing Your Body's pH Factor*, as the best ways of improving your energy levels, based on all the things I've tried and researched.

The focus of Dr Guerrero's book, and Tony Robbins' 'Pure Energy Live' seminar, is all about the importance of maintaining a healthy acid-alkaline pH balance in the body, and that unhealthy pH levels are at the root of all diseases. This is based on the original research about the acid alkaline balance that was done by Dr Neil Solomon many years ago at Johns Hopkins University.

## Maintaining a Healthy pH Balance in your Body

It is critically important that the body maintains a blood pH level of 7.36, or as close to that level as possible, which is slightly alkaline. The delicate acid-alkaline balance is important, not only for the health of the body, but also for the level of energy you have available. It's so important that your cells and your organs would literally shut down if the level was to vary by one or two points.

The pH level in our biochemistry is necessary to allow for the tiny electrical pulses to occur, i.e. for all the nerves being able to send signals via the tiny pulses of electricity. All the cells and all the organs of the body need to have this electrical power in order to be energised, which is required for them to be completely healthy and to be functioning efficiently.

The delicate pH level of the blood is also important because the outside of a blood cell has to have a negative charge. This negative charge stops the blood cells from clumping together.

If the blood cells lose the negative charge then they start to stick together and will therefore start going through the bloodstream more slowly. This degradation will mean that less oxygen is going through the bloodstream and can significantly impact your energy levels. Also if the blood cells start clumping together too much then they may not even be able fit through some of the tiny capillaries throughout the body.

But the challenge is that nowadays diets tend to be way too acidic, and the body constantly has to compensate to deal with all the excess acid. Because if the bloodstream and the environment inside the body becomes too acidic then it will interfere with the negative charge of the blood cells, and they will not only weaken but will die. When they die they release their own acids into the bloodstream, which compounds the problem.

When there is too much acidity the body has to compensate by using its alkaline reserves to neutralize the acid, or it stores excess acid in the fat reserves. But if you're constantly consuming an overly acidic diet, day after day, and putting more and more strain on the alkaline reserves, then over time the body exhausts the alkaline reserves and has to start leeching calcium from your bones.

When you're continually consuming an overly acidic based diet you're also creating an environment where Candida yeast can proliferate, i.e. creating a Candida albicans infection. These yeasts mercilessly eat through you glucose supply in your bloodstream, which not only takes nutrients away from the body, but also negatively effects your energy levels.

The Candida yeast infection can also start to break down your soft tissues and start eating your proteins. And just to make things even worse the Candida yeast also excretes its own waste and their waste is acidic, which is just continuing to add to the problem.

# Cleansing and Alkalising

To help flush out the build up of acidity in the body there is a need to cleanse the system by focusing your dietary habits onto much more alkaline based foods. Just to give you an idea it takes 4 parts of alkalinity to balance out, or neutralise 1 part of acid.

In the section below I list some of the alkaline based foods, but it can mostly come from having a big salad and a green 'super foods' based drink each day, and from increasing your consumption of green vegetables, particularly green leafy vegetables and broccoli.

Green vegetables are not only extremely high in alkalinity but they're also among the highest in terms of the electrical energy they can provide to the body. They provide around 70 to 90 megahertz of energy. Raw almonds are also alkaline and provide 40 to 50 megahertz, so they're ideal for snacking on.

The super greens drink made from the green powder is between 250 and 350 megahertz.

I typically have a big salad for lunch each day. My personal favourite is the Waitrose Bright & Crunchy Rainbow Salad or the simple M&S classic salad, but there are plenty to choose from in all the supermarkets. I also drink 1 heaped teaspoon of the Next Gen U Organic Super Greens Powder mixed with a pint of water each day. The Next Gen U Organic Super Greens Powder is available on Amazon (https://smile.amazon.co.uk/Next-Gen-SuperGreen-Supplement-Supergreens/dp/B07BCK824F) and contains the following ingredients: Barley Grass, Chlorella, Wheat Grass, Acai Berry, Flax Seed, Baobab, Guarana, Maca and Matcha.

Tony Robbins also has his own branded Bioenergy Greens drink available if you're based in the USA (https://store.tonyrobbins.com/products/bioenergy-greens).

As well as the super greens drink, I also drink 1 heaped teaspoon of the Naturya Organic Wheatgrass Powder mixed with a pint of water each day. The Naturya Organic Wheatgrass Powder is also available on Amazon (https://smile.amazon.co.uk/dp/B004RODLTC) and in some supermarkets too. But wheatgrass is one of the most potent so you may need to gradually build up to taking that every day if your diet has been very acidic for many years.

You generally want to be drinking plenty of water to help aid with the cleansing process. Ideally mineral water or at least filtered tap water, I often add freshly squeezed lime or lemon juice into the water too, which you might think is acidify but is actually alkalising to the body.

I've experienced significant improvements in my energy levels since changing my dietary habits to being much more alkaline in nature. Nowadays my diet is made up of a lot more salads and a lot more green vegetables, plus the super greens drink and wheatgrass drink.

These dietary changes really helped to turn my constant lack of energy around, but please be aware the improvements came gradually, little by little. It was almost imperceptible. I didn't suddenly start feeling better on day 1. And it wasn't until I stopped and thought, hang on a minute, I've actually got some energy now and am feeling so much better, that I noticed things were really working. And so I stuck with the changes and gave my body chance to heal. I became much more active, exercising daily, and feeling much better, and because of that, found it much easier to stick with a rock-solid sleep routine and rock-solid sleep hygiene.

## Acidifying and Alkalising Foods

In his book, *In Balance for Life: Understanding and Maximizing Your Body's pH Factor*, Dr. Alex Guerrero describes in detail the importance of the acid-alkali balance. He also provides meal plans and lists of foods that are acidifying and foods which are alkalising.

Alex explains the following regarding acidifying and alkalising foods:

*"Once they are digested and metabolized - literally burned down - all foods leave a residue of ash in your body. Depending on the type of food and its mineral content, the ash residue is either acidic or alkaline. Foods that produce an acidic ash have an acidifying effect on the body, and therefore lower pH levels. Foods that leave an alkaline ash have the effect of raising pH levels.*

*It is important to note that the acidifying or alkalising effects of the foods you eat are far more significant, in terms of your health, than the foods' inherent pH values prior to their consumption. For example, a number of foods that are acidic in nature, such as certain citrus fruits and vinegars, actually have a strongly alkalising effect on the body after they are digested and metabolised. Not all acidic foods are acidifying when they are eaten, nor are all alkaline foods alkalising when consumed."* (77)

And:

*"Acidifying foods are generally high in proteins, carbohydrates, and/or fats. Such foods include:*

*Alcohol*
*Milk and other dairy products*
*Breads*
*Poultry*
*Caffeine products (chocolate, coffee, black tea)*
*Refined and processed foods*
*Commercial condiments*

*Seeds and nuts (except for almonds and Brazil nuts)*
*Fish*
*Soda*
*Certain grains*
*Sugar and artificial sweeteners*
*Legumes*
*Tap water*
*Meats*
*Yeast products"* (80)

And:

*"Alkalising foods are rich in alkaline minerals and contain little or no acidic substances. In addition these foods produce no acidic ash when they are digested and metabolized, regardless of the amount consumed at any meal. Foods in this category include:*

*Alkaline mineral water*
*Certain nuts (almonds and Brazil nuts)*
*Certain fruits (bananas, grapefruit, lemons, limes, avocados, and tomatoes)*
*Sprouts (such as sprouting alfalfa, chickpeas and mung beans)*
*Cold-pressed oils*
*Vegetables*
*Herbs, spices and salts"* (86)

I highly recommend switching out some of the Acidifying foods and replacing with Alkalising foods where feasible.

The body is very good at dealing with an overly acidic diet up to a point, but if it's been going on for years and years and years, then eventually by the time you hit your late 30s and

40s and later you're really going to start paying the price health-wise and with the significant impact on your energy levels and your body's ability to fight off infection.

## Other Sources

Coupled with the recommendations from Dr Alex Guerrero's book and the Tony Robbins '*Pure Energy Live*' seminar in his '*Get The Edge*' audio program, I also used some of the suggestions from the books, *How Not to Die: Discover the Foods Scientifically Proven to Prevent and Reverse Disease*, and the *How Not to Die Cookbook*, by Michael Greger MD and Gene Stone. In '*How Not to Die*' they go into details about all the scientifically proven benefits of a plant-based whole-foods diet. It reinforces what Dr Alex Guerrero talks about in his book, but it comes at it from a completely different angle.

I did try sticking with a purely vegan diet for a while and then a vegetarian for a long while especially with a focus on consuming more alkaline based foods. Nowadays I have re-introduced some meat back into my diet, but I'm using the suggestions from the book, *Eat Right 4 Your Type*, by Dr Peter D'Adamo. It's a great book because it explains why humans have evolved to have different blood types; and it lists loads of foods that are beneficial for each of the different blood types, and which foods should be avoided. It also provides a 10-day plan for each blood type.

For each blood type, Dr D'Adamo, lists the problem foods to avoid for Lectin Sensitivity; Liver Detox Dysfunction; Hyperassimilator Tendencies; and Imbalanced Microbiome. He also lists super-foods for each blood type which help to block Lectin Sensitivity; Build Active Tissue Mass (enhances carbohydrate metabolism, helps with weight loss); Improve Liver Function; Blunt Hyperassimilator Tendencies; and Balance Microbiome (increases microbiome diversity, discourages microbial imbalance).

Dr Peter D'Adamo also provides cookbooks specifically for each of the different blood types, which are also helpful when looking for ideas for your new dietary habits.

However I highly recommend detoxifying and alkalising first before and sticking with much more alkaline based diet before introducing more of the acid based foods back.

## Getting Tested

Rather than just blindly following the suggestions in the books, I also had a food intolerance test done and discovered that wheat was a major red flag for me. And sugar, chocolate, tea and coffee were warning flags. That was a bummer as they were among the top ingredients in many of the things I had previously consumed. For example, my lunches previously consisted of sandwiches, baked goods, chocolate, tea or coffee. And for my evening meals I'd often have pasta with meat and a sugar-rich sauce or a pizza. But after some perseverance and a little testing on myself, because I was sceptical, I did find that sugar and wheat were pretty big energy destroyers for me. Yeah you'd get an initial boost, but it was the killer energy dips that sapped me of the precious energy reserves, and I got a lot of headaches as well.

So, for me, reducing my sugar intake and switching more to a whole-foods plant-based diet with a focus on consuming much more alkaline based foods, and then later on including some other foods based on the 'blood type' diet had a big impact. It helped reduce the killer dips in energy, and as a side benefit I lost a little weight too.

Cutting out wheat also seemed to reduce the headaches. And after I'd been on these dietary changes for a while, I discovered that I no longer needed to take the antihistamine tablets for hay fever. I was able to cut them out altogether and found that my symptoms of hay fever are significantly reduced. From what I've learnt, this seems to be related to an intolerance to wheat, but may also be related to general food sensitivities and the inflammation they can cause in the body.

I also haven't had a single cold since adopting a much more alkaline based diet. In previous years I would seem to catch all the coughs and colds going around especially from my children, and would feel extra rough as a result. But I literally haven't caught a single cold since. I've still been out and about, and on flights and in contact with lots of people, same as before, but my body now seems to be so much better at fighting off any infections.

# Making the Change

Significantly reducing sugar intake is a tricky one though, because sugar is in just about everything and if you're used to having a couple of chocolate bars a day and a donut and some cake and sugar in your hot drinks, then cutting it out is tough.

All the dietary changes and especially cutting out sugar is one step where I recommend going easy on yourself. If you're currently having a chocolate bar every day, cut back to half a bar per day for 1 week, and then to one small square per day the next week, and then finally eliminate it altogether. The same goes with cakes and biscuits and any other sugary snacks and drinks.

If you're tired of being tired all the time, and your energy levels are shot to pieces already, I highly recommend adopting the principles described in Dr Alex Guerrero's book and in Tony Robbins' 'Get the Edge' program and cutting out the sugar and switching to the whole-food, plant-based diet, coupled with the guidelines in 'Eat Right 4 Your Type'. But be careful to cut foods out and introduce the changes gradually. And give your body chance to heal and stabilise those all important energy levels. It's also likely to take a while before you start noticing any benefits.

One of the other benefits I noticed with the improved dietary habits, as I've mentioned, is that I very rarely get headaches now. Which is obviously a good thing, but worth noting because it was particularly helpful when going through the weeks of stopping all napping and sticking with the strict sleep hygiene. Because when I tried to stick with that in earlier years, before the dietary changes, I would always suffer from an increase in headaches and it would make it that much harder to stick with a rigid sleep hygiene routine, e.g. I might have to take headache tablets containing caffeine or try to face a difficult night with a headache. The dietary changes significantly helped to remove this potential obstacle.

As with any dietary program it is recommended to seek guidance from your doctor and/or nutritionist before proceeding.

## Typical Dietary Habits

Just to set the scene, prior to sorting out my dietary habits, I would typically have something like the following for breakfast: Cereal, toast, fruit juice, cup of tea with milk and sugar.

Mid-morning snack: crisps, or breakfast bar and another cup of tea.

For lunch I'd typically have: ham sandwiches, crisps, pastries, a chocolate bar and a cup of tea with milk and sugar.

Mid-afternoon snack: a chocolate bar, snack bars, pastries, and/or biscuits, and then more tea throughout the day.

For dinner, I might have: spaghetti Bolognese, or pepperoni pizza, or pasta with meatballs, fried chicken with rice, or pie and chips, or a ready meal.

I've got nothing against these foods. I used to live on them, literally. The problem, I discovered, was that I have an intolerance to most of the items listed. Wheat in particular, but also sugar, chocolate and caffeine. And, according to Dr. D'Adamo in *'Eat Right for Your Type'*, it's advisable for my blood type to avoid the kind of meats I'd been consuming on a daily basis.

These foods are probably fine for a short period of time, but over years and years, they gradually build up toxins in the body, creating low and unstable energy. And as Tony Robbins describes in *'Get the Edge'* it's all acid based; very little alkaline based foods.

I also drink plenty of water these days instead of all the tea. This not only helps to ensure I'm well hydrated throughout the day, but also helps to flush out the toxins that have built up over the years.

So it doesn't take a genius to realise that over a long period of time, these two different sets of dietary habits are going to have vastly different results. And that's exactly what happened. My energy levels significantly improved, my overall feeling of well-being improved, I also just generally look healthier. People I haven't seen in a long time always comment that I'm looking very well. Maybe they're just being polite, but I do feel a whole lot better, so that's what really counts here.

When I started on the dietary changes, I thought I'd miss all my favourite foods, and that I wouldn't be able to stick with the plan. Yes, it was hard for the first 2 days (but only the first couple of days were a slight challenge, getting used to the new foods). Once I'd got used to it, I really didn't miss any of the things I previously ate, which genuinely surprised me. Well, actually, I must admit I missed one thing: I missed aromatic crispy roast duck and plum sauce from the Chinese takeaway, which we used to have quite often. So after a while, I would still have some crispy duck, but only rarely. But other than that, I really didn't miss anything, and I have absolutely no desire to go back to what I ate before. In fact it would probably make me sick now.

And to loop back to the main reason for this book... feeling good and having significantly improved energy levels all massively helped to resolve decades of sleep maintenance insomnia. It's like my body was getting back into a natural balance. Everything fell into place... finally!

Could I have fixed my sleep without sorting out my dietary habits? I really, really tried, but for me, I just don't think it was possible. Having that belief now is more than enough to keep me on the right path, health wise, and sleep routine wise. Would I go back to my old dietary habits now? As my 4-year-old often says "No way!"

It was a challenge, changing my dietary habits for the first few days, but I soon found, to my surprise, that I didn't miss many of the foods I'd consumed before. And once I started to feel the benefits I was hooked on sticking with the changes.

The other important thing I do is not over-eat at any one meal. We've all stuffed ourselves to the point of bursting, usually on Christmas day. But what resulted? Massive amounts of afternoon napping and snoring. Your body needs a lot of energy to process and digest so much food, so over-eating can also be a killer for sapping energy reserves. I seem to work best by eating smaller portions and having healthy snacks in between. So I'd recommend keeping portion sizes to sensible levels to help maintain your all-important energy levels.

Here's an example of my typical daily routine now:

Up around 5:45am (by the way I still don't need an alarm - I wake early - I set an alarm for the latest time just in case, but I don't stay in bed waiting for it if I'm already awake), make the bed, clean teeth, wash face. Drink a pint of water with freshly squeezed lemon or lime juice.
6:10am Exercise either out walking (if nice weather) or on the exercise bike.
7:00am shower.

7:15am breakfast (usually omelette with steamed kale + super greens drink).

7:35am school run.

8:30am work.

10:30am mid-morning snack, which is usually something like almonds, walnuts, live culture yogurt, apple, grapes, grapefruit, along with a cup of green tea.

12:00pm lunch (salad with fish in extra virgin olive oil, or soup).

3:00pm snack again (similar to mid-morning snack).

3:30pm school run.

5:00pm dinner (vegetables with meat/fish/sweet potato).

5:30pm time with kids.

7:30pm snack + pint of water with wheatgrass powder

8:00pm free time together with girlfriend (watching TV / movies / reading / learning).

10:00pm up to bed.

Not all days are the same of course. Things crop up. Sometimes I can go out walking at different times and walk further (depending on other commitments and work schedules). Sometimes I find I've slept longer, which is great - I don't force a fixed hard time for waking, but there won't be too much variation there. I know it's highly unlikely I'm suddenly going to sleep in an extra 2 hours one day.

Another typical day is something like...

Up around 6:00am, make the bed, clean teeth, wash. Drink a pint of water with freshly squeezed lemon or lime juice.

6:15am Exercise weights/toning.

7:00am shower.
7:15am breakfast (usually omelette with steamed kale + super greens drink).
7:30am free time with a cup of green tea.
8:30am time with kids.
10:30am snack.
12:00pm lunch (salad with fish, or soup, or vegetables with lamb or fish).
1:00pm out for a walk (2 hours).
3:00pm snack.
3:30pm time with family.
5:00pm dinner (vegetables with meat/fish/sweet potato).
5:30pm time with kids.
7:30pm snack + pint of water with wheatgrass powder
8:00pm free time together with girlfriend (watching TV / movies / reading / learning).
10:00pm up to bed.

Basically there's flexibility there, but I aim to do some exercise every day, ideally in the morning. And eat healthy foods with healthy snacks in between. Food choices are guided by details mentioned earlier. And with the aim of being active in the day time and/or engaged in tasks / activities I can really get fully absorbed into.

Bloody hell you live like a monk, I hear you cry! Do I completely restrict my dietary choice? No. Do I eat cake? Yes, sometimes. Do I eat ice cream? Yes, sometimes. Same goes for chocolate. Will I drink a cup of tea or a chocolate milkshake? Yep, sometimes. But I don't consume them every day, just very rarely. Basically, I don't feel it's restricted. I'm happy with the routine and love the better sleep, energy and health. Also, I'm more attuned to noticing when things have sapped my energy or what might have caused a headache to occur, which is rarely the case nowadays.

Worried about the meals being inconvenient at lunch time? Try this: salad bowl + tin of sardines in olive oil. Add the sardines into the salad bowl including all the olive oil. The olive oil mixes well with the salad and the fish helps to make the salad tasty. It takes literally 30 seconds to make. For an added boost you could also add in a spoonful of flaxseed and a small sprinkling of pink Himalayan sea salt.

For some added taste and variety I can also recommend adding some spoonfuls of the M&S Supergreen Salad, which contains a mix of cucumber, edamame beans, apple, broccoli, courgette, sugar snap peas, pumpkin seeds, spinach and coriander, with an apple, soy and ginger dressing. It's delicious and healthy and it's available in small 176g packs or in large 600g packs for serving 6-8 people.

In some ways I should be thankful to my insomnia because it has forced me to search to find answers to better health and vitality.

Just as an aside, if you are interested in dieting then there's a simple sure-fire way of shedding weight. You don't need to count the calories, you don't need to watch portion sizes, you don't need all the low fat garbage (actually your body needs the good fat), and you don't even need to exercise excessively. All you need to do is to significantly reduce your consumption of refined carbohydrates and alcohol. Refined carbohydrates (or simple carbohydrates) include sugars, white flour, pasta, pastries, white bread, pizza dough, white rice, sweet desserts, and many breakfast cereals. And replace them with plenty of veggies and planet-based whole-foods. If you care at all about your health it's well worth taking a careful look at your consumption of refined carbohydrates.

# Exercise

Just as important as the dietary improvements is regular exercise. Not only does it oxygenate your whole system, if helps to filter all the chemicals your body would rather get rid of. You also get more exposure to sunlight, which helps with maintaining the body's natural sleep-wake cycle and you're becoming fitter and healthier in process.

It doesn't need to be anything massively strenuous and ideally needs to be in the morning, rather than the evening. For me, personally, I found that walking every day really helped improve my sleep at night. I now walk for approximately one and half hours each morning whenever possible. Walking is an easy, gentle exercise. I'm also fortunate enough to have an exercise bike at home, so if the weather is particularly unpleasant then I can still get the exercise at home using the exercise bike.

Of course, you could build on this, firstly by making it a brisk walk for a few days, then, if you really feel like it, breaking into a jog. I realise that this is different and that you'd need the right clothes and footwear, so it's not quite the same as going for a walk every day, but jogging is quite addictive. Once you're into it, you soon won't find walking anywhere near enough. With your change of diet, you'll also have more energy, so it becomes a win-win situation.

If you are interested in running I recommend checking out Stu Mittleman's book *Slow Burn: Burn Fat Faster by Exercising Slower*. Stu Mittleman is an ultra-endurance racer who ran 1,100 miles in 10 days, and regularly competes in the 1,000-Mile World Championship races. What's particularly interesting is that Stu doesn't seem to have energy shortage problems on these extreme races!

It's highly unlikely that we'll want to be running such colossal distances, but what's useful is that in his book, Stu explains exactly how to train at a level that's comfortable for your current level of fitness and age - based around heart-rate ranges. He even goes into details about choosing the right training shoes and maintaining the right posture. The important point is that you're training at a comfortable level specifically aimed at slowly burning through much longer lasting fat stores rather than rapidly burning through your sugar reserves. Stu explains that most people are usually exercising too intensely, or too quickly, which can result in pain and discomfort and feelings of nausea. And he states that training too intensely is not the way to build the most efficient system of energy consumption.

Stu also goes into in detail about maintaining the right nutritious diet, focusing on a bias towards alkaline based food, echoing many of the points described by Tony Robbins. This all loops back to significantly improving your energy levels on a consistent basis.

But, if you're not keen on running, I stress that walking on a daily basis is just as beneficial for your health, well-being and helping to reinforce and optimise the all important sleep-wake cycles.

# Products That Didn't Work

I've included this section here as a reference on some other things I tried when trying to improve my constant lack of energy, but which didn't work for me. Maybe they're of interest to you, but based on my experience I'd say you don't need them unless specifically directed to use them by your nutritionist.

**L-Tyrosine Extra Strength, Amino Acid, 50 Veggie Capsules by Vita Premium**
https://www.amazon.co.uk/gp/product/B01FZJDS90/
According to Wikipedia (June 2020):
>*"Tyrosine or 4-hydroxyphenylalanine is one of the 20 standard amino acids that are used by cells to synthesize proteins. It is a non-essential amino acid with a polar side group.*

*Tyrosine is a precursor to neurotransmitters and increases plasma neurotransmitter levels (particularly dopamine and norepinephrine), but has little if any effect on mood in normal subjects. However, a number of studies have found tyrosine to be useful during conditions of stress, cold, fatigue (in mice), prolonged work and sleep deprivation, with reductions in stress hormone levels, reductions in stress-induced weight loss seen in animal trials, and improvements in cognitive and physical performance seen in human trials."*

I read about L-Tyrosine in Dr. Jacob Teitelbaum's book: *"From Fatigued to Fantastic: A Clinically Proven Program to Regain Vibrant Health and Overcome Chronic Fatigue and Fibromyalgia"*. For me personally, I didn't notice any effect while taking the L-Tyrosine capsules other than having slightly looser stool than usual.

To learn more about Tyrosine I recommend reading Dr. Jacob Teitelbaum's book: *"From Fatigued to Fantastic: A Clinically Proven Program to Regain Vibrant Health and Overcome Chronic Fatigue and Fibromyalgia"*.

**Enzymatic Therapy, Fatigued to Fantastic - Energy Revitalization System**, Berry Splash Flavour (609g)
https://www.amazon.co.uk/gp/product/B0013OX5DQ

Ingredients:
- Vitamin A (55% as beta carotene and as retinyl acetate) - 4,500IU - 90% (DV)
- Vitamin C (ascorbic acid) - 500mg - 833%
- Vitamin D (as cholecalciferol) - 1,000IU - 250%
- Vitamin E (as mixed tocopherols) - 30IU - 100%

- Vitamin K (as phytonadione) - 100mcg - 125%
- Thiamin (as thiamin HCl) (vitamin B1) - 75mg - 5,000%
- Riboflavin (vitamin B2) - 75mg - 4,412%
- Niacin (as niacinamide) - 50mg - 250%
- Vitamin B6 (as pyridoxine HCl) - 45mg - 2,250%
- Folate (as Folic Acid and Quatrefolic® brand (6S)-5-methyltetrahydrofolate glucosamine salt) - 400mcg - 100%
- Vitamin B12 (as methylcobalamin) - 500mcg - 8,333%
- Biotin - 200mcg - 67%
- Pantothenic Acid (as calcium d-pantothenate) - 50mg - 500%
- Calcium - 80mg - 8%
- Iodine (as potassium iodide) - 200mcg - 133%
- Magnesium (as magnesium aspartate) - 200mg - 50%
- Zinc (as zinc gluconate) - 15mg - 100%
- Selenium (as L-selenomethionine) - 55mcg - 79%
- Copper (as copper gluconate) - 500mcg - 25%
- Manganese (as manganese citrate) - 2mg - 100%
- Molybdenum (as sodium molybdate) - 125mcg - 167%
- Sodium - 20mg - <1%
- Potassium (as potassium citrate) - 136mg - 5%
- Whey Protein (milk) - 5.5g
- Malic Acid - 1g
- Betaine - 750mg
- Inositol - 750mg
- Inulin (from chicory root) - 750mg
- Taurine - 500mg
- Glycine - 390mg
- L-Tyrosine - 377mg
- N-Acetylcysteine (NAC) - 250mg
- L-Serine - 240mg

- Stevia Leaf Extract - 150mg
- Choline Bitartrate - 100mg
- Grape Seed Extract standardized to 85% polyphenols (42.5 mg), including procyanidolic oligomers (PCOs) - 50mg
- Boron (as sodium borate) - 2mg

This is a very good quality product and you're not likely to find more vitamins packed into a single supplement. I tried this for approximately 2-months, following the suggested daily dosages. I'm sure it was doing some good, but unfortunately I didn't notice any improvement in energy levels while taking the Energy Revitalization System powder.

**Muscleform D-Ribose ATP Fuel** 100% pure powder - 650g
https://www.amazon.co.uk/gp/product/B00DL0VGNQ
I didn't notice any effect while taking the Muscleform D-Ribose powder.

To learn more about D-Ribose I recommend reading Dr. Jacob Teitelbaum's book: *"From Fatigued to Fantastic: A Clinically Proven Program to Regain Vibrant Health and Overcome Chronic Fatigue and Fibromyalgia"*.

## Summary

Having researched quite a number of health and diet related books while on the quest to find ways of significantly improving my energy, I thought it worth summarising some of my findings and finally, the key things that I found worked best for me.

The various books don't all line up and agree on all points as you'd expect, and it can be a bit confusing to know what things to go for. However, there was general agreement on following the common sense things, which I thought worth summarising here:

1) Vegetables are king, especially green leafy vegetables.

2) Unsaturated fats (monounsaturated and polyunsaturated fats) are beneficial - more commonly referred to as 'good fats'. Beneficial unsaturated fats include foods such as avocados, olive oil, nuts, salmon and sardines.

3) Trans fat are harmful and to be avoided - more commonly referred to as 'bad fats'. Just to give you an idea, French fries, doughnuts, deep-fried fast foods, cookies, cakes and pastries all usually contain trans fat.

4) Cut down on processed food as much as possible.

5) Cut down on sugar as much as possible.

There were a couple of other recommendations that cropped up more often than not, which were:

6) Saturated fats are to be used sparingly. Foods such as palm oil, whole milk, cheese, butter and ice cream.

7) The 'Mediterranean diet' is a popular example of a balanced healthy diet.

There's some disagreement with regards to whether eating meat is healthy or not, similar to some of the debates in society at present. Some books say meat is harmful to your health and best avoided, whereas other books say it's necessary for a balanced diet but that not all meats are necessarily good for you. That's one of the reasons why I particularly liked Dr D'Adamo's book *'Eat Right 4 Your Type'*, which includes specific meats in the lists of foods that are good and which are not so good for each of the different blood types.

There's also some disagreement on fruits as well, interestingly enough. Some books say you can eat as much fruit as you like and if you overeat on fruit it will just go straight through you. Other books say eating too much fruit causes spikes in blood sugar levels and therefore some moderation is best. But all books agree that some fruit should be included as part of a healthy balanced diet. I've found that eating too much fruit in the morning will cause my energy levels to spike but then take the unwanted nosedive soon after, so they're not ideal for maintaining optimal consistent energy levels. But I do eat a small selection of fruits on a daily basis, which again is guided based on the fruits most beneficial for my particular blood type and with the most alkalising affect.

I've tried being a vegan, but I found it quite challenging to rigidly stick to it on a continual basis. I've tried being a vegetarian for quite a long while and did feel a lot better on that compared to my old dietary habits, however I appreciate it is entirely possible to still make bad dietary choices while being a vegetarian. Based on my own personal experiences I feel the best fit for me has worked out as being a bias towards a whole-food, plant-based diet, particularly loaded with alkaline based foods and with plenty of water, but also including some specific meats based on recommendations for my specific blood type from Dr D'Adamo's book, especially fish.

But the biggest bang for the buck came initially from the cleansing and alkalising as described in Tony Robbins' *'Get the Edge'* audio program and covered in Dr Alex Guerrero's book, *In Balance for Life: Understanding and Maximizing Your Body's PH Factor Understanding and Maximizing Your Body's PH Factor*. After the initial cleansing phase, it's all about maintaining a sensible balanced diet that's rich in alkaline, plant-based whole-foods and which promotes your health, vitality and that all important abundance of energy.

Anyway, enough details on healthy eating; this book is all about resolving chronic insomnia. Is it possible to resolve chronic insomnia without improving or making any changes to your dietary habits? In many cases it probably is. But if you've been suffering with insomnia for many, many years and you've tried everything and nothing seems to be working, then shifting your focus to improving your energy could be the key that also breaks you out of the vicious cycle. It certainly was for me and in the process I became a whole lot healthier too.

The next challenge is trying to get my kids to eat healthily. Although my teenage son said he wished someone could hypnotise him into liking salad, so maybe there is hope yet!

# Chapter 7

## Getting Back to Sleep

I'm sure most people have been there... lying awake at night, tossing and turning and being unable to get to sleep, or get back to sleep. For anyone suffering from sleep maintenance insomnia, it's a nightly occurrence, and when the problem has been there for many years, night after night, it's easy for the feelings of despair to creep in and make the already challenging situation a whole lot worse.

So what can we do while we're working through the sleep hygiene and lifestyle changes and persevering to get our sleep in a much better state? We're clear on the fact that it's likely to take some time before our sleep is fixed, probably a few weeks. And there will probably be some bad nights along the way, even the occasional bad night once your sleep is in a much better place. It's 'normal' to have an occasional bad night. Personally I don't want any more bad nights, but that goal might be too much of a stretch!

Before I finally found the answer, it felt like I was continually being robbed of the precious four hours extra sleep, which I felt I desperately needed, especially during the years when I blamed everything on poor sleep.

## Why We Wake in the Night

There are many theories out there about why we might wake up in the early hours. Here are just a few I've come across over the years:

**Segmented (Polyphasic) Sleep**: This is where your night is split into two separate periods of sleep. You'd sleep for several hours, wake for a couple of hours and then sleep again for the second phase of sleep. Historians believe that this way of sleeping is how humans naturally evolved, such as the work by Roger Ekirch. And there is some belief that the time awake in-between the two phases is apparently a very creative period.
https://www.sleepadvisor.org/segmented-sleep/

**Chinese medicine "body clock"**: In Chinese medicine there is a belief that waking at the same time every night could signify a problem with a specific organ in the body depending on what time you wake each night, for example waking at 3am every night could indicate Liver Qi stagnation.

I actually tried a course of acupuncture specifically for treating sleep maintenance insomnia. Sadly in my case it had absolutely no noticeable effect as I described in an earlier chapter.

**Hypothalamic sleep-centre suppression**: this is getting into technical medical knowledge that is a bit beyond me. Putting it at my level of understanding... complex biological stuff happens in the hypothalamus relating to the release of hormones to regulate the sleep wake cycle. Things can potentially disrupt that biological process, such as fibromyalgia, which can result in early morning waking.

I've added a section at the end of this chapter with more details about the Hypothalamus and how it relates to insomnia.

For more information specifically about fibromyalgia or chronic fatigue syndrome or if you'd like to learn more about hypothalamic sleep-centre suppression then I recommend reading *"From Fatigued to Fantastic: A Clinically Proven Program to Regain Vibrant Health and Overcome Chronic Fatigue and Fibromyalgia"* by Dr. Jacob Teitelbaum.

If you'd like to learn more about the role of the hypothalamus and it's possible affects on sleep then I recommend reading *"Hormones in Harmony: Heal Your Hypothalamus for Optimal Health, Graceful Aging, and Joyous Energy"* by Deborah Maragopoulos. Some details from Deborah's book are provided in the Hypothalamus section below.

**Hyperthyroidism**: An overactive thyroid (hyperthyroidism) can cause anxiety and insomnia including both problems falling asleep and problems with waking up frequently during the night.

**Adrenal Fatigue**: when the adrenal glands aren't functioning efficiently and therefore not producing hormones at optimal levels then insomnia can occur. This can cause both sleep maintenance and sleep onset insomnia.

Please see the sections in the next chapter for details regarding the Thyroid and Adrenals and how they relate to insomnia.

**Sleep apnoea**: I'm not going to cover sleep apnoea in this book, but if you suspect you might have sleep apnoea then you definitely need to see your doctor and get a referral to have that treated as soon as possible.

**Depression, stress, anxiety**: all can cause the early morning waking and being unable to get back to sleep.

**Low blood sugar levels**: When blood sugars drop too low this apparently can cause early morning waking.

I've tried eating all manner of foods before bedtime that are suggested to help keep blood sugar stable throughout the night, such as boiled eggs, avocadoes, nuts, cheese & crackers, celery sticks with hummus, but alas that also didn't help in my particular case. I've tried drinking nothing in the evening and only in the morning and early afternoon. Unfortunately that also didn't help in my case.

**You might be going to bed too early:** If you're going to sleep at 9pm it wouldn't be at all surprising if you're waking at 3am or 4am, which is around 6 or 7 hours sleep. And, by the way, this includes if you're falling asleep in the evening while watching TV. If you're nodding off around 9pm on the sofa before going to bed, then that really counts as when your sleep time is starting.

**Other medical problems:** Some on-going medical problem causing pain or discomfort, such as acid reflux, which can sometimes cause you to wake feeling nauseous when you've been asleep for a few hours. I don't personally suffer from this, but for those of you readers who do, my chapter on the dietary changes for improved energy could help you a lot.

We may never really know for sure why exactly we keep waking up in the early hours. Maybe in the distant future, when our bodies have armies of medical nano-bots monitoring every bodily function, we might know for sure. But until then, we just may never know the root cause.

## How to Get Back to Sleep

Knowing the reason why we wake up in the early hours is all very interesting, but what's really important is how-the-devil do we get back to sleep in those precious hours before we need to be up.

Lying awake in the early hours, tossing and turning and being unable to get back to sleep is the major pain point for anyone suffering with sleep maintenance insomnia, especially if the problem has been there for many years, night after night.

Part of my problem was that my mind would be off at a hundred miles an hour almost as soon as I realised I was awake. Trying to quiet the mind just seemed to make it race even more. I tried all the tricks including the variations on counting down or up. My thoughts would still come racing along even in the gaps between the numbers I was counting. I could even have thoughts simultaneously darting about while stoically focusing on my breathing. Eventually, after an hour or so, I would give up and miserably get out of bed for a couple of hours.

I would also over-analyse things, such as 'ooh I wonder how this latest product, pill, remedy (or whatever I was trying at the time) was working'. And of course all that thinking would just prolong the time I was lying wide awake.

Or just as I felt I was about to nod off, my mind would leap up and go 'but what about that mistake you made 5 years ago', or 'what about that embarrassing situation you had 10 years ago', or 'what about this terrible thing that might happen'! Great, now it feels like I'm never going to sleep. And on, and on it would go, night after night.

Over the years I tried all manner of different tricks, tips, techniques and strategies to try and get a little more sleep before having to start the day. Most of the things didn't really help much, some of which you've seen listed before, but the following tips have been most helpful in my particular case:

**Change the whole situation from being a negative thing to being a positive thing.** I'm not talking about the mind games here, where you just have to 'let go' and 'not worry about it', etc, which I've always completely failed at. What I mean is a complete paradigm shift in how you feel and think about this situation.

For years I would feel such frustration, anger and sometimes even despair about the constant early morning waking. It would be a constant source of anxiety for me and I would feel so bitter about always losing those precious hours of sleep every single night. By the way, all those bad feelings are completely natural - we humans have evolved to think more negatively than positively (primitive man: is that a rock or a lion - better to think it's a lion, etc.) - but all those bad feelings and negative thoughts are not at all helpful in this situation and just push sleep further away.

It wasn't until I'd almost given up trying to fix my sleep and just sort of accepted that I was going to be awake for several hours and might as well do something, that things became easier and I was able to get back to sleep a little earlier and easier than before.

It doesn't happen very often these days, but when it does, I now see the 'early hours awake' time as productive 'me' time. I get some quality time to myself while everyone else is still asleep. It's peaceful, it's quiet and it can be an incredibly creative and valuable time if you're not suffering with too much brain fog. This is a far better and more productive way of feeling and thinking about the situation, and you tend to feel more relaxed as a result. Thus sleep doesn't get pushed away so much.

**Related to that is getting out of bed for a while.** After many years of this unwanted, torturous experience, I knew without fail that I would be awake for several hours. Just lying in bed, not sleeping would end up making me feel frustrated and push sleep further away. And would result in negative associations with being in bed. So, for me, I've found it is usually better to get out of bed and do something that isn't overly stimulating.

This is about seeing it as productive 'me' time (within the conditions of not being overly stimulating). I wouldn't recommend playing Grand Theft Auto, learning to dance hip-hop, or playing the bagpipes (unless you live alone in a remote location). So what are some of the things I got up to in the wee small hours? Here are a few examples:

**1) Learning a language:** I worked on learning vocabulary for a foreign language. I didn't watch online lessons, but instead would use lists and books I had already prepared and simply went through the rote task of learning the vocab. This was very effective at getting me to feel sleepy again and had the benefit of making feel like I'd achieved something and of course distracted me from focusing on negative unhelpful thoughts.

**2) Reading:** I got through a great many books, thanks to these extra hours. I would recommend actual paperback or hardback books rather than e-book editions, so you're not reading on an electronic device. I'd also avoid intense thriller type books, or riveting page turners, which could keep you awake and/or reading for longer.

I'd get through quite a lot of business and technical books, which are sometimes quite dry in nature and often quite effective at inducing the feelings of sleepiness again.

**3) Affirmations:** I tried 'affirmations' for a while. I'm a fairly logically chap - being a computer programmer and all - and 'affirmations' seemed a little bit airy-fairy at the start. But I'm reasonably open-minded and believe in the power our thoughts have. So I stuck with it for several months and found it to be helpful at directing my thoughts to more positive things and generally to get me feeling sleepy again. It did however remind me of having to write lines as punishment for stuff when I was school, but other than that it was worth a try.

If you're not familiar with affirmations, it is basically about writing and/or saying, over and over again some positively stated phrases about what you'd like to achieve, change or improve about yourself, but written in the present tense, as if you'd already achieved, changed or improved that thing. It's useful to have some affirmations that start with the two very powerful words "I am..." For example, you might write out a whole page of lines something like "I am full of health, energy and vitality" or "I am creative" or "I am lucky." Affirmations can also be helpful for countering the usual negative type "I am..." things we can sometimes tell ourselves on a daily basis without even realising it, such as "oh I am so clumsy," or "I am always failing at this."

I'd avoid being overly fanciful and far-fetched with the affirmations because your mind is likely to be thinking 'yeah, right' as you're writing out the lines.

If you're into this kind of thing and would like to learn more about affirmations then I can recommend checking out 'The "I AM" Discourses', Saint Germain Series of books. They're spiritual in nature but have some good ideas on affirmations for creativity, protection, intelligence and abundance, etc.

**4) Sketching:** I tried sketching and colouring. I wanted to learn to do the manga style drawings. That was a laugh at first. My young kids could have done a better job. I was eventually able to draw something sort of resembling a manga style character, after getting through several notebooks. But in the end, I found colouring to be more relaxing, but I didn't feel it was productive.

**5) Writing and journaling:** Updating my journal with thoughts and ideas is a daily habit I still stick with now. I will jot down all manner of things with no particular formatting in mind. Some of the things I write down include possible ideas for new software, websites, blogs, books, business ventures, etc. This helps to get the ideas out of your head and onto paper, so you're not continually trying to remember stuff in the middle of the night.

**6) Programming:** Sometimes, if I really felt the creative urge, or had the answers to some technical problem waiting in my mind, I would program. Partly to get it done and out the way, so my mind wouldn't keep going over it, but also just to go with that particular feeling. But I have f.lux installed on my computer to reduce blue light glare and would always wear my blue light blocking glasses.

But I'd recommend minimising the use of electronic equipment, as the exposure to light is counterproductive to getting back to sleep.

Other ideas for things to try could include writing poetry, sketching, creating a comic book, writing, doing a jigsaw, even craft work.

If you feel you're wide awake and you know from painful experience that you're going to be awake for a long while, you might want to get out of bed for a while and try some of the tips above. Find something relaxing and potentially productive. But it's important to see it as useful 'me' time, and not to let the feelings of frustration and annoyance wash over you. Then when you start to feel sleepy again you can return to bed.

So you return to bed and still have one or more hours of possible sleep before you need to be up to start the day. Hopefully you're feeling sleepy again and the feelings of frustration, anger and despair are no more. If you're not feeling sleepy yet, then go back to the previous step.

So how do you actually get back to sleep... these are the tips that have helped me:

**Wear earplugs:** sleep in the early morning is typically lighter sleep from my experience and there are likely to be more noises, such as traffic starting to build up, car doors, bird songs, etc. I am easily disturbed during light sleep, so for me, earplugs are useful at this time.

**Stay cool but not cold:** sometimes I feel quite hot when getting back into bed, so I kick the duvet off sufficiently to feel cool but comfortable.

**Relax and breathe:** Get into your usual sleep position, get comfortable, relax your jaw and other facial muscles, and start to breathe a bit more deeply and slowly than normal. On some out-breaths, feel yourself relaxing into the bed and pillow more and more. Just be with the feelings and enjoyment of the relaxation and feelings that you can do absolutely nothing. Now you can just rest. This is still your 'me' time, but it's a chance to simply relax and do absolutely nothing.

**If you sleep, great.** But if you don't sleep, don't fret. Just allow that time for your body and eyes to get some extra rest.

Just continue to maintain the deeper, slower breathing and don't move around too much.

If your mind does start racing and you're having trouble calming your thoughts, I found that shifting my focus to more relaxing calming thoughts helps to distract from what could otherwise easily turn into a blizzard of unwelcome and unhelpful thoughts. Here are a few suggestions to consider while still continuing with the deeper, slower breaths:

**Focus on gratitude.** Think of what things you can be grateful for in your life. Even being grateful for the many things we take for granted such as having a bed, the sheets, the curtains, taps with running water, food, clothes, the list can easily get very long when you start to think about it.

**Focus on finally have chance to rest:** I would also think about how happy I am to finally be in bed, which is where I'd wanted to be most of the day when feeling so tired. For example, 8 hours ago, all you wanted to do was curl up in bed. Now you finally *can* curl up in bed. Get absorbed in the feelings of finally being in bed, able to rest and relax.

**Visualise:** Remember a time when you felt completely relaxed and then stay with that feeling. For me, this is a time when I was on a sun lounger, the weather was pleasantly warm, there was a clear blue sky, it was quiet and I was just watching some birds circling high in the sky above.

If you can't remember any time when you felt really relaxed, just invent a scenario in your mind. Maybe it could be on a beach, or at home, or in a spa, or a hammock. Whatever works best for you. It's all about calming and enjoying the relaxation.

**Another tip to consider:** during the day time I keep a simple journal, where I note down thoughts, ideas, useful information and events that I want to remember. It's generally useful because I can look back when needed, but it also helps to stop my brain trying to remember stuff at night time.

There are many other ideas available on online, such as the blog post, 10 Ways to Tame Your Monkey Mind and Stop Mental Chatter: https://daringtolivefully.com/tame-your-monkey-mind.

Nowadays, I still occasionally wake in the middle of night, usually for a pee, but then I go back to sleep again. I also still wake early, but not at 2am or 3am, as I did before. These days I usually wake around 5:30am or 6am, which I go with, and use as part of my daily routine.

## Mindfulness and Loving-Kindness

Some other things that I've found to be particularly helpful are the practice of mindfulness and loving-kindness. These can really help to reduce the endless chatter in the mind and can significantly improve feelings of happiness and a sense of well-being and calm.

Loving-kindness is very simple and very powerful. It focuses the attention away from oneself and onto other people instead. This really helps to calm the mind and significantly decreases the unhelpful negative mental chatter that the ego likes to generate. For example, all the judging of oneself and others, complaining, condemnation, stereo-typing and many other negative thought patterns that can often cloud our minds.

This is how it works: Several times throughout the day randomly identify people, for example people you might drive past, people in your office building, people on the bus, people who walk past you or who are waiting in line somewhere. And secretly wish for them to be happy. The key word here is 'secretly'. Just simply think to yourself, "I wish for that person to be happy." That is all you need to do. Don't say or signal in any way that you have done this; it's purely a short thinking exercise. It's so quick and simple that you can do it many times per day. I recommend just once or twice per hour is more than enough.

Try it for a few days and see what happens. Notice how you feel and how little things start to change for you.

It is also something you can do in the night if you're lying awake for a long time. Think of different people in turn and wish for them to be happy. Visualise the person in your mind and wish for him or her to be happy.

The practice of loving-kindness really seems to disarm and halt the ego in its tracks and dissolves a lot of the unhelpful mental chatter. And you just generally feel happier and more at ease.

As well as the practice of loving-kindness, I also recommend the regular practice of mindfulness.

I learnt a lot about mindfulness from the works of Eckhart Tolle. In particular I highly recommend reading the books *"The Power of Now: A Guide to Spiritual Enlightenment"* and *"A New Earth: Create a Better Life"* both by Eckhart Tolle.

Mindfulness involves bringing your full attention to whatever activity you're engaged in at the present moment. For example if you're making a coffee bring your full attention to the simple act of making a coffee. If your mind starts drifting back to thinking about the things you need to do, or things that have gone wrong, or how poorly you slept, etc. then notice this and gently bring your full attention back to the activity you're engaged in. In the simple act of making a coffee you can also think about, and feel gratitude for, all the many people and steps involved in getting the coffee beans from the field to your kitchen.

Or if you're talking with a friend, colleague or family-member, be fully present for that conversation. Give the person your full attention.

The more you can fully focus on the present moment the more powerful the experience. I remember one time that really stands out to me... I was watering the garden and bringing my full attention, appreciation and wonderment to the plants and flowers I was watering. My mind was still and I was completely absorbed in the simple act of watering the garden, and for the briefest of moments I felt an incredible peace and joy come over me and a short burst of laughter escaped from my mouth completely involuntarily. It was a really powerful experience, hard to describe, but has made me a big believer in mindfulness and the power of the present moment.

## Breaking Free of Repetitive Negative Thought Patterns

If you find that you're continually going over the same unhelpful negative thought patterns, for example if you've recently suffered a split in a relationship, or someone has broken the trust you had for them. And these thought patterns just seem to go on and on and you really want to reduce them and stop the powerful hold they have over your mind, then the following 'eye scramble' technique can be helpful.

You're going to think I'm a bit crazy with this one as it feels a bit ridiculous, but I promise it works. Whenever you catch yourself going over the negative thought patterns that you want to end, you immediately start humming a song to yourself, such as happy birthday, while at the same time moving your eyes about into different positions!

The act of moving the eyes around and humming happy birthday to oneself completely interrupts the negative thought pattern.

I learnt about this technique from the excellent "Charisma on Command" YouTube channel, specifically from the "Why You Don't Feel Good Enough" video: https://www.youtube.com/watch?v=gcH6tFugYfo

You probably want to avoid doing this in front of your boss or while paying for groceries at the checkout, but definitely worth trying at appropriate times.

## Summary

I sincerely hope that if you stick with the recommendations in this book you too can enjoy significant improvements in the quality of your sleep and won't have all the extra hours of 'awake time' to play with. But I feel I should re-iterate: this is a gradual process. It can take time to resolve decades of broken sleep. So while you're working through the sleep hygiene, diet and lifestyle changes, and persevering until your sleep is in a much better state, you can use the tips suggested above as ideas on what to do when you're lying awake for long periods in the early hours.

The practice of mindfulness and loving-kindness will also help calm the mind and bring a powerful sense of peace and acceptance to your life.

If, once in a while, I do still wake in the night, or way too early, then I use the steps and tips described above. The key point here is that it will no longer be plaguing your mind all day, and no longer be such a source of anxiety and worry. I'm no longer reading quite so many books, but I can definitely live with that trade off.

# Chapter 8

## Hypothalamus, Thyroid and Adrenals

The sections that follow provide some details on some specific reasons about why we might be waking in the early hours and suffering with long term insomnia.

What I find interesting is that if you read a book about the hypothalamus it clearly states that problems with the hypothalamus can cause insomnia, among many other things. The same is also true with the thyroid and with the adrenals.

For example, in Deborah Maragopoulos' book '*Hormones in Harmony: Heal Your Hypothalamus for Optimal Health, Graceful Aging, and Joyous Energy*', she describes how the hypothalamus orchestrates your entire endocrine system (all your hormones) and your sleep cycles, among many other things. And she describes:
"*Whether you have trouble falling asleep, staying asleep, or both, you have a dyscircadian rhythm.*

*"Insomnia is often initiated by stress. But chronic insomnia is an imbalance of you day/night cycle - your circadian rhythm. Your hypothamalmus controls your circadian rhythm. If you can't sleep at night, your hypothamalmus is out of balance."* (90)

In Dr. James L. Wilson's book '*Adrenal Fatigue: The 21st Century Stress Syndrome*', he states: "*When the adrenals are not secreting the proper amount of hormones, insomnia is also one of the likely outcomes.*" (9)

In Dr. Barry Durrant-Peatfield's book '*Your Thyroid and How to Keep it Healthy: The Great Thyroid Scandal and How to Survive it The Great Thyroid Scandal and How to Survive It*', he states: "*Insomnia is a common complication; and thyroid supplementation may, between 2 and 3 weeks, restore normal sleeping.*" (59)

And yet possible problems, or low-functioning, of the hypothalamus, thyroid and/or the adrenals never seems to get mentioned in any books specifically about insomnia. It's like you either have a well-known condition such as sleep apnoea, restless leg syndrome, narcolepsy or sleep walking, etc. Or you have plain old vanilla insomnia and need to be treated with some form of CBT. There seems to be no middle ground, which is a bit of hole in my opinion.

The same can also be true when discussing problems with insomnia with your GP. For example, I once asked my doctor if my chronic insomnia could be caused by hypothalamic sleep-centre suppression and he just looked at me blankly and immediately dismissed it. I think they may have to ensure you go through all the usual sleep hygiene and a CBT course before exploring other options.

But if you've been religiously sticking with bullet-proof sleep hygiene and all the other recommendations in the CBT programs for months on end and yet still have poor sleep, then it might very well be a problem with the hypothalamus, thyroid and/or the adrenals.

In all three of these cases it is advisable to find yourself a good, qualified, nutritionist who can advise you on the best course of action for your particular case. It's also important that you get the dietary changes, as described in Chapter 6, in place and well established before starting on any course of supplements. This will help to ensure your body is better able to absorb and utilise all the good stuff in the supplements, and to ensure you're not just feeding a Candida yeast overgrowth.

That might have been why many of the other supplements I tried in the past didn't work very well for me, because the environment was too acidic inside my body and with too much Candida and because I was self-navigating without any guidance from a nutritionist.

In the sections below I'll briefly cover some details and recommendations specifically for healing the hypothalamus, thyroid and the adrenals.

# Hypothalamus

The hypothalamus is a small region of the brain, located near the pituitary gland. It plays a crucial role in the release of hormones and in maintaining daily physiological cycles, along with other important functions. When the hypothalamus isn't working properly there are a whole range of conditions that can occur, from the mild to the life-threatening. And there are a whole range of different symptoms that could signal a hypothalamic problem, including insomnia.

So, how do we repair imbalances in the hypothalamus? This is where I'm going to recommend following the advice in Deborah Maragopoulos' book 'Hormones in Harmony: Heal Your Hypothalamus for Optimal Health, Graceful Aging, and Joyous Energy'. It's a very informative and easy to understand book describing the role of the hypothalamus in simple terms; what can cause it to stop working properly; what symptoms can occur when it's out of balance; and how to get it back into balance.

Deborah explains:

> "The hypothalamus does not know the difference between a tiger chasing you and you being late for work. The adrenal response is the same: Adrenaline -> Cortisol -> DHEA. Over and over and over again, day after day, week after week, for months, maybe years on end, the stress on modern day life puts a toll on the adrenals. Eventually they become fatigued, producing less and less cortisol and DHEA until you can hardly function." (75)

124

And:

> *"Profound fatigue - You struggle to wake up in the morning. You need caffeine and sugar to start your day. Your energy crashes in the afternoon. Sometimes you get a second wind at night and cannot sleep. This is a reversed circadian rhythm and it's usually early in the course of adrenal dysfunction."* (75)

Deborah's book also covers some details about her Genesis Gold® powder based supplement, which is very good stuff. The only downside is that the shipping costs from the US to the UK are quite expensive when you include the custom charge (applicable at the time of writing).

I've been taking the Genesis Gold® supplement each morning for several months now and it may very well have also helped with the improvements to the quality of my sleep alongside the other dietary and lifestyle changes I had made.

But, as with the other changes, it takes time for the benefits of regularly taking the Genesis Gold® supplement to be fully realised. For example, Deborah advises:

> *"Many nutrients are used in multiple locations in your body. For example the amino acids - serine, cysteine, arginine - are used in your brain... but they're also used in your gut.*
>
> *If your gut is deficient, then all of it will be used there first, meaning that your sleep might be disturbed, your brain is foggy, you feel kind of moody. All of which will improve, but you need to be patient while your body heals from the inside out."* (subscribed email)

As well as the powder based supplement there are also hypothalamus glandular extract supplements available from a variety of suppliers. These supplements contain dried and ground-up animal glandular tissues or extracts of those tissues. These supplements can help to support the hypothalamus. It's not something I've tried, but in any event it's definitely worth consulting with a nutritionist before proceeding with any such glandular extracts.

# Thyroid

The thyroid gland is an endocrine, hormone-producing, organ located in your neck. It is one of the most important glands in the body as it controls the rate at which the various organs and systems function. It has an effect on many things throughout the body including metabolism, energy levels, circulation and sugar regulation.

An underactive thyroid (hypothyroidism) can cause fatigue and excessive drowsiness. An overactive thyroid (hyperthyroidism) can cause anxiety and insomnia including both problems falling asleep and problems with waking up frequently during the night.

The thyroid is linked to the adrenal glands, therefore when there are problems with the thyroid the adrenal glands can also become imbalanced. Problems with adrenal glands can have an impact on the release of cortisol, which effects sleep. If thyroid hormones are out of balance, the adrenal glands can produce too much cortisol, making it difficult to drop off to sleep. And when the body is stressed, cortisol is released by the adrenal glands. This hormone tells the body it is time to be alert and wake in the morning, but this can also happen in the night time causing difficulties in falling back to sleep.

In Dr. Barry Durrant-Peatfield's book '*Your Thyroid and How to Keep it Healthy: The Great Thyroid Scandal and How to Survive it The Great Thyroid Scandal and How to Survive It*', he describes many of the symptoms that can occur when there are problems with the thyroid; what can cause problems with the thyroid; and various treatment plans.

One possible cause of imbalances is past trauma that may have impacted the thyroid. In his book, Dr. Durrant-Peatfield states:

> "*Thyroid Trauma: This means that the thyroid gland, exposed as it is, may be subject of damage from the outside. One obvious example here is whiplash injury. Something like 30% of people who suffered whiplash injury have been found to develop hypothyroidism. Another obvious one is somebody getting you by the throat; and over vigorous examination has also been cited as a cause. Stretching the neck, as for example, banging your chin on the dashboard in a car crash, is another one.*" (49)

I suffered a heavy blow to the chin when I came off my bicycle at about the age of 13 while whizzing down a hill. I landed hard on my chin, partially ripped open my labial frenum (the soft tissue between the bottom gum line and the lips) and caused hairline fractures in the jaw bone. This may very well have also caused some trauma to my thyroid which may well have been a possible cause of my sleep problems, or the initial trigger point for the start of insomnia.

Dr. Durrant-Peatfield also explains:

> *"Failing sleep patterns, especially in older people, and those due to stress and anxiety, may be restored by melatonin. All patients have reported improved sleep, using the average dose, 3 mg at night. But it can be used with great effect in the prevention of jet lag, basically speeding up (or slowing down) the body's own adjustments. You take your melatonin before bedtime, at your new destination. If you wake up, repeat the dose."* (105)

And:

> *"Not only are very many depressed people actually hypothyroid and therefore easily treated without antidepressants, but also there are other disturbances of brain function that can be and often are the result of lowered metabolic activity. Cognitive loss and memory loss are common complaints - this is the 'brian fog' familiar to so many. Concentration, attention span, the ability to think quickly and the ability to memorise things, all become degraded. Until you have the benefit of thyroid supplementation, you may be unaware of what you're missing. You may not have realised that you weren't enjoying life as perhaps you deserve. (Poor sleep is another problem which quietly puts itself right)."* (187)

There are a whole range of different treatments recommended in Dr. Durrant-Peatfield's book depending on the range and severity of symptoms. These include the use of melatonin before bedtime and again if you wake in the night as noted in the excerpt above. But again this is where you need to get some guidance from your nutritionist on the best course of action for your particular case.

# Adrenal Fatigue

The adrenal glands are endocrine organs that secrete hormones directly into the bloodstream. They are small triangle shaped glands located on top of each kidney. The adrenal glands make hormones that are essential for body functions, including the steroid hormone cortisol.

If you're continually feeling stressed day after day, and you're always feeling overtired or run down, then you might be overtaxing your adrenals and could therefore be suffering from what's known as Adrenal Fatigue, which is increasingly recognised as a common source of extreme tiredness.

It's possible that Adrenal Fatigue Syndrome is the root cause of prolonged feelings of fatigue along with other symptoms such as brain fog, a general difficulty in concentrating, anxiety, an inability to lose weight or allergies.

Also, insomnia can be caused by Adrenal Fatigue, but also the adrenals can be fatigue by chronic insomnia. It's like it feeds on itself making things worse!

In her book 'Hormones in Harmony: Heal Your Hypothalamus for Optimal Health, Graceful Aging, and Joyous Energy', Deborah Maragopoulos states:

*"The longer you're in deep REM sleep, the more energy you have during the day. That's because your adrenal glands need to rest at night in order to fuel your daytime activity. Adrenal fatigue is a result of chronic insomnia."* (93)

When the adrenals are constantly working overtime due to stress, they become so over-taxed, eventually they start to fail leading to a raft of symptoms.

In his book *'Adrenal Fatigue: The 21st Century Stress Syndrome'* Dr James L. Wilson explains the following:

*"Sleep is very important to full adrenal recovery but the twist is that sleeplessness is sometimes one of the signs of adrenal fatigue."* (124)

And:

*"There can be several reasons for sleeplessness with adrenal fatigue. If you're waking between 1:00 and 3:00am, your liver may be lacking the glycogen reserves needed for conversion by the adrenals to keep the blood glucose levels high enough during the night. Blood sugar is normally low during the early morning hours but, if you are hypoadrenic, your blood glucose levels may sometimes fall so low that hypoglycemic (low blood sugar) symptoms wake you during the night. This is often the case if you have panic or anxiety attacks, nightmares, or sleep fitfully between 1:00 and 4:00am. To help counteract this have one or two bites of a snack that contains protein, unrefined carbohydrate, and high quality fat before going to bed, such as half a slice of whole grain toast with peanut butter or a slice of cheese on a whole grain cracker.*

*"Both too high and too low nighttime cortisol levels can cause sleep disturbances."* (125)

If you suffer with any of the symptoms mentioned above and/or you think Adrenal Fatigue might be one of the possible causes of your sleep problems then it's well worth discussing this with your nutritionist. They'll likely start you on a course of Magnesium supplements and/or adrenal glandular extracts.

I can recommend the 'Nutri Advanced Nutri Adrenal Extra Tablets' (https://www.nutriadvanced.co.uk/nutri-adrenal-extra-60-tabs.html), which contain hormone-free glandular extracts of both the adrenal and pituitary glands (bovine source from New Zealand), along with the following:

Vitamin C (ascorbic acid)
Pantothenic acid (d-calcium pantothenate)
Vitamin B1 (thiamine HCl)
Vitamin B2 (riboflavin)
Vitamin B6 (pyridoxine HCl)
Vitamin B3 (niacinamide)
Magnesium (citrate)
Zinc (ascorbate)
Chromium (picolinate)
Bioflavonoids
Choline (bitartrate)
Adrenal concentrate
Pituitary

These tablets will need to be taken before 11am each day, but you need to be guided by your nutritionist on this.

# Summary

For those of whom it may not be plainly clear to see, this is my first ever attempt at writing a book. Thank you for buying my book and taking the time to read it. I sincerely appreciate the time you've invested and I sincerely hope it has been useful to you in some way, and I hope this book has convinced you that what might have seemed like irresolvable chronic insomnia can actually be resolved, even if it's been a persistent pest for many, many years. Following my recommendations will take patience, perseverance and some discipline, but the tides of weariness can be washed away and the curse of insomnia can be conquered.

Here's a brief summary of all the steps I used to overcome decades of broken sleep:

1) Ensure your sleep environment is as optimal as possible.

2) Maintain impeccable sleep hygiene.

These first two requirements are the foundations for helping to ensure you have the best chance of a good night's sleep.

On their own they won't resolve decades of broken sleep, but they can't be neglected.

3) No napping.

4) Maintain a consistent routine even at weekends.

There's no getting around these two requirements for resolving decades of broken sleep. Technically they're part of maintaining impeccable sleep hygiene but I've listed them as separate points as they can be the most challenging to continually stick with, especially after a run of bad nights, but they're essential for helping to reset your body's natural rhythms.

5) Follow the suggestions in chapter 7 on Getting Back to Sleep, especially if you're lying awake for long periods each night.

6) Practice mindfulness and loving-kindness.

These will help while sticking with the new routine on the road to improving your sleep.

7) Follow the dietary suggestions in chapter 6 to alkalise and energise.

8) Shift your attention away from sleep and onto improving your energy levels, health and feeling good.

These last steps are really important. They will help you to regain your energy levels, boost your sense of well-being and reclaim your passion for life. In turn, that will significantly help you to have the strength to stick with impeccable sleep hygiene and the new routine, and really importantly, help you to worry much less about sleep. Fix your energy, feel good and let sleep take care of itself.

If you'd like more information or would like to get in touch please head over to my website at longroadtosleep.com. I will endeavour to keep it up to date with any new information and will try to reply to all reasonable requests and enquiries.

I wish you well on your quest in overcoming insomnia. Stay strong, stay committed and above all sleep well!

# Bibliography

Amen, Daniel G., and Amen, Tana. *The Brain Warrior's Way: Ignite Your Energy and Focus, Attack Illness and Aging, Transform Pain into Purpose.* Penguin Random House LLC, 2016.

Amen, Daniel G. *Feel Better Fast and Make It Last.* Tyndale House Publishers Inc., 2018.

Barone, Daniel. *Let's Talk about Sleep.* Rowman & Littlefield, 2018.

Chaitow, Leon. *Candida Albicans: The Non-Drug Approach to the Treatment of Candida Infection.* Thorsons, 2003.

Chopra, Deepak. *Boundless Energy: The Complete Mind-body Programme for Overcoming Chronic Fatigue.* Random House, 1995.

Chopra, Deepak. *Restful Sleep: Complete Mind-body Programme for Overcoming Insomnia.* Random House, 1994.

Cousins, Norman. *Head First: The Biology of Hope and the Healing Power of the Human Spirit.* Penguin Books, 1989.

D'Adamo, Peter. *Eat Right 4 Your Type: Fully Revised with 10-day Jump-Start Plan*. Penguin Random House UK, 2016.

Diamond, Harvey, and Diamond, Marilyn. *Fit for Life*. Bantam Books, 2004.

Durrant-Peatfield, Barry. *Your Thyroid and How to Keep it Healthy: The Great Thyroid Scandal and How to Survive it The Great Thyroid Scandal and How to Survive It*. Hammersmith Press Limited, 2006.

Ferriss, Timothy. *Tools of Titans: The Tactics, Routines, and Habits of Billionaires, Icons, and World-Class Performers*. Vermilion, 2016.

Galland, Jonathan, and Galland, Leo. *The Allergy Solution: Unlock the Surprising, Hidden Truth about Why You Are Sick and How to Get Well*. Hay House, 2016.

Gariti, James, and Breese, Terri. *Tired of Being Tired? The Doctor Will See You Now*. 2012.

Germain, St. *The I AM Discourses*. 1965.

Greger, Michael, and Stone, Gene. *How Not To Die: Discover the foods scientifically proven to prevent and reverse disease*. Macmillan, 2016.

Greger, Michael, and Stone, Gene. *The How Not To Die Cookbook: Over 100 Recipes to Help Prevent and Reverse Disease*. Macmillan, 2017.

Guerrero, Alex. *In Balance for Life: Understanding and Maximizing Your Body's pH Factor*. Square One Publishers, 2005.

Hay, Louise L. *You Can Heal Your Life*. Hay House UK Ltd, 2005.

His Holiness the Dalai Lama, and Cutler, Howard C. *The Art of Happiness: A Handbook for Living*. Coronet, 1999.

Idzikowski, Chris. *Sound Asleep: The Expert Guide to Sleeping Well*. Watkins Media Limited, 2013.

Lam, Michael, and Lam, Dorine. *Adrenal Fatigue Syndrome: Reclaim your Energy and Vitality with Clinically Proven Natural Programs (Dr. Lam's Adrenal Recovery Series)*. Adrenal Institute Press, 2012.

Maragopoulos, Deborah. *Hormones in Harmony: Heal Your Hypothalamus for Optimal Health, Graceful Aging, and Joyous Energy*. Best Seller Publishing, 2016.

Meadows, Guy. *The Sleep Book: How to Sleep Well Every Night*. Orion Books Ltd, 2014.

Mittleman, Stu. *Slow Burn: Burn Fat Faster by Exercising Slower*. Harper, 2001.

Myss, Caroline, and Shealy, C. Norman. *The Creation Of Health: The Emotional, Psychological, and Spiritual Responses That Promote Health and Healing*. Bantam, 1999.

Hanh, Thich Nhat. *The Miracle Of Mindfulness: The Classic Guide to Meditation by the World's Most Revered Master*. Rider, 2008.

Newport, Cal. *Deep Work: Rules for Focused Success in a Distracted World*. Paitkus, 2016.

Riha, Renata L., and Anne Helena Rennes, Editor. *Sleep: Your Questions Answered*. DK, 2007.

Robbins, Anthony. *Get the Edge: A 7-Day Program To Transform Your Life*. Robbins Research International Inc., 2000.

Robinson, Ken. *Finding Your Element: How to Discover Your Talents and Passions and Transform Your Life*. Penguin Books, 2013.

Robinson, Ken. *The Element: How Finding Your Passion Changes Everything*. Penguin Books, 2009.

Stephens, Sasha. *The Effortless Sleep Companion: From chronic insomnia to the best sleep of your life*. Dark Moon Ltd, 2013.

Stephens, Sasha. *The Effortless Sleep Method: The Incredible New Cure for Insomnia and Chronic Sleep Problems*. 2010.

Stevenson, Shawn. *Sleep Smarter: 21 Essential Strategies to Sleep Your Way to a Better Body, Better Health, and Bigger Success*. Hay House UK Ltd, 2016.

Teitelbaum, Jacob. *From Fatigued to Fantastic: A Clinically Proven Program to Regain Vibrant Health and Overcome Chronic Fatigue and Fibromyalgia.* Penguin Books Ltd, 2007.

Tolle, Eckhart. *The Power of Now: A Guide to Spiritual Enlightenment.* Hodder and Stoughton, 2005.

Tolle, Eckhart. *A New Earth: Create a Better Life.* Penguin Random House UK, 2016.

Walker, Matthew. *Why We Sleep: The New Science of Sleep and Dreams.* Scribner, 2017.

Wilson, James L. *Adrenal Fatigue: The 21st Century Stress Syndrome.* Smart Publications, 2001.

Winter, Chris W. *The Sleep Solution: why your sleep is broken and how to fix it.* Penguin Random House LLC, 2017.

Printed in Great Britain
by Amazon